MEDICAL CARE
AT THE END
OF LIFE

MEDICAL CARE

AT THE END

OF LIFE

A Catholic Perspective

DAVID F. KELLY

GEORGETOWN UNIVERSITY PRESS
Washington, DC

IN MEMORY OF MY FATHER,

Martin J. Kelly,

KILLED IN ACTION IN FRANCE, NOVEMBER 9, 1944

As of January 1, 2007, 13-digit ISBN numbers will replace
the current 10-digit system.
Paperback: 978-1-58901-112-0

Georgetown University Press, Washington, D.C.

Library of Congress Cataloging-in-Publication Data

Kelly, David F.
  Medical care at the end of life : a Catholic perspective / David F.
Kelly.
       p.   cm.
  Includes bibliographical references and index.
  ISBN 1-58901-112-0 (pbk. : alk. paper)
  1. Medical ethics—Religious aspects—Catholic Church.   2. Medical
care—Religious aspects—Catholic Church.   3. Medicine—Religious
aspects—Catholic Church.   I. Title.
  [DNLM: 1. Terminal Care—ethics.   2. Catholicism.   WB 310
K295m   2006]
  R725.56.K46   2006
  174.2—dc22

                                        2006003017

Printed in the United States of America

This book is printed on acid-free paper meeting the requirements of the American
National Standard for Permanence in Paper for Printed Library Materials.

13 12 11 10 09 08 07 06   9 8 7 6 5 4 3 2
First printing

CONTENTS

ACKNOWLEDGMENTS

I WISH first to acknowledge the essential role played by the St. Francis Health System, a multi-institutional system of hospitals and nursing homes owned and run by the Sisters of St. Francis of Millvale, Pennsylvania, and to the remarkable people who worked there prior to its closing for financial reasons in 2002. Without my work at St. Francis this book could not have been written. The people of St. Francis welcomed the discussion of ethics and welcomed me; they were patient as I tried to learn what real hospitals were about. I especially acknowledge John Hoyt, director of critical care medicine and chair of the ethics committee. It was he who hired me for the sabbatical I took at the hospital in 1989 and 1990 and then arranged for me to continue as a staff ethicist.

Duquesne University and its people have been equally important in supporting this book and the work that led up to it. The university gave me a sabbatical grant to write *Contemporary Catholic Health Care Ethics*, and while on sabbatical, I did most of the work for this book as well. I am thankful to the Duquesne administration, to Michael Slusser, chair of theology, and to present and past deans, provosts, and presidents. They have recognized that medical ethics needs both theory and practice and have been greatly supportive of Duquesne's Health Care Ethics Center. I am grateful to Aaron Mackler, colleague in the Theology Department and associate director of the Health Care Ethics Center, who took over the administration of its graduate degree programs while I wrote. He also read the previous book and the major additions to this one, making suggestions for improvement.

INTRODUCTION

FOR the past thirty years I have written about medical ethics and taught the subject to physicians, nurses, social workers, hospital chaplains, undergraduates, and graduate students. During this time I have been active in American hospitals and nursing homes, helping patients and their families deal with the difficult and often painful issues regarding medical treatment at the end of life. As I have worked on hospital ethics committees, designed hospital and nursing home policy, and taken part in ethics consultations, I have also helped my own friends, colleagues, and family members work their way through these issues. In this book I write about what I have learned. My aim is to provide patients, their families, hospital chaplains, and the entire health care community with a useful resource for thinking about decisions that so many people, at some point in life, must face.

This, then, is a practical guidebook that describes in detail the American ethics and law about forgoing treatment. It draws on Roman Catholic medical ethics, since much of what has become American policy in the area was taken from Catholic sources, and it engages certain questions that are currently debated within Catholic medical ethics. But it is not intended only or even primarily for those interested in Catholic issues. It is a book about the ethics of end-of-life care in America.

Two recent events have focused attention, both within and without the field of Catholic bioethics, on this critical issue. In March 2004 Pope John Paul II delivered an allocution, also known as a formal speech, concerning nutrition and hydration (John Paul II 2004). And then, more recently, came the case of Theresa Marie Schiavo, the Florida woman whose feeding tube was removed after years of political and legal dispute. I will discuss both of these events, given the profound implications they have had within Catholic bioethics and on the American medical and political landscape.

There are eight chapters in this book. The first five develop in detail the bases for what I call the "American consensus" on forgoing treatment. Chapter 1 introduces the three pillars, or bases, for the American approach to this area and presents the first of them: the widespread agreement that some life-sustaining treatment is ethically optional and may be withheld. Chapter 2 details the important distinction between actively killing dying people and allowing them to die, a distinction I call the second pillar. Chapters 3, 4, and 5 analyze in detail the third pillar, the important legal and ethical issues of who decides and how the decision is made, including issues concerning competent and incompetent patients as well as advance directives (living wills and durable powers of attorney for health care). I introduce the *Schiavo* legal case in this context.

Chapter 6 is about feeding tubes. I discuss and reject the proposals of some who, by requiring nutrition and hydration for permanently unconscious patients, would undermine the claim that treatment is optional if its burdens outweigh its benefits. Here I again note *Schiavo* and discuss at some length the 2004 papal allocution. In chapter 7 I reject arguments by those who would support the practice of euthanasia and physician-assisted suicide and would reject the claim that there is an important difference between killing and allowing to die. And in chapter 8, on medical futility, I confront claims by those who would reduce the authority of patients to make decisions about their treatment.

This book is not meant to be an exhaustive treatment of end-of-life matters. It is intended to highlight what I believe to be the most important issues at stake—issues that require clear thinking and some understanding of medical ethics and relevant legal cases. I can only hope that readers of this book will gain some useful knowledge, and some degree of comfort, from my efforts.

ABBREVIATIONS

CPR	cardiopulmonary resuscitation
DNR	do not resuscitate
DPA	durable power of attorney
DRG	diagnosis related group
ER	emergency room
HMO	health management organization
ICU	intensive care unit
IRB	Institutional Review Board
PAS	physician-assisted suicide
PDE	principle of double effect
PET	positron emission topography
PSDA	Patient Self-Determination Act
PVS	persistent vegetative state
UDDA	Uniform Definition of Death Act
USCC	United States Catholic Conference

—☙ *Chapter 1* ❧—

Ordinary and Extraordinary Means

F ROM the 1960s to the 1980s, Americans were unable to reach a consensus on the morality of forgoing medical treatment. Scholars disagreed about many of the issues—this continues today, as we will see—the basic stance of U.S. law had not been determined, the medical profession was largely unsure of what to do, and hospital policies varied widely. To the degree that there was a general approach, it was usually that the physician decided what to do in each individual case, and often that decision was to insist on ongoing aggressive treatment even when there was little human benefit. In the 1960s and 1970s, the growing field of bioethics reacted against this approach, against what came to be called "medical paternalism" (Veatch 1973). This criticism and other factors resulted in a radical change, so that by the 1990s it was possible to speak, at least in some sense, of an American consensus. This consensus emerged from bioethical scholarship and showed itself in a number of significant court cases, starting with the *Quinlan* case in 1976 and continuing through the U.S. Supreme Court cases on physician-assisted suicide (PAS) in 1997; it was also the result of a number of important decisions reached by governmental committees and commissions. It is true, of course, that there has never been universal agreement on the issues, and today what consensus exists is under attack, especially from those who would legalize euthanasia and/or PAS and, to a lesser extent, those who would use "medical futility" to reduce the decision-making authority of patients and surrogates and return it in some degree to physicians. The consensus is also under attack from those who claim that certain treatments, particularly medical nutrition and hydration (feeding tubes), are morally required even when their benefit to patients is slight or nonexistent, as in the case of patients in a persistent vegetative state. I will discuss all of these issues in detail in later chapters. Yet despite these areas of controversy, it is possible to speak of a consensus in U.S. law, medicine, and ethics about the legal and ethical rightness of forgoing life-sustaining treatment.

THE THREE PILLARS OF THE CONSENSUS

The best way to understand the current consensus is to see it as based on three pillars of support. The first pillar is the recognition that not all treatments that prolong biological life are beneficial to the patient. In the Catholic tradition, this concept is expressed in the distinction between ordinary and extraordinary means of preserving life, the topic of this chapter.

The second pillar is the agreement that there is a moral difference—and ought to be a legal difference—between killing (active euthanasia) and allowing to die. This will be the topic of chapters 2 and 7.

In the U.S. legal system, these two ethical bases have been combined with a basis in law, the legal concept of the right to autonomy, privacy, and liberty. This is the third pillar, which will be developed in chapters 3, 4, and 5. Taken together, these three pillars provide the foundation on which the present consensus concerning the moral and legal rightness of forgoing treatment has been built.

The first two of these pillars are well established within the Roman Catholic tradition, which had already developed, prior to the arrival of so-called American bioethics in the 1960s and 1970s, a detailed and complexly argued system of medical ethics. The only other tradition, religious or secular, to have done this is Jewish medical ethics, and that tradition, for various reasons that need not concern us here, has had a lesser impact on American secular medical ethics and American law than has the Catholic tradition. Indeed, it is probable that the current consensus would have been impossible had these concepts not already been developed in Catholic moral theology.

ORDINARY AND EXTRAORDINARY TREATMENT

The first pillar on which the current consensus is based is the general agreement that not all medical treatment that prolongs biological life is of benefit to the patient. Thus some life-sustaining treatment can be forgone.

The ethical distinction between mandatory and optional treatment has been provided by the Catholic tradition in its centuries-old distinction between "ordinary" and "extraordinary" means of preserving life, terms often used even in secular conversation and policies. The distinction goes back at least to the sixteenth century, was included in the important work of Alphonse Liguori in the eighteenth century, and was emphasized and made popular by the teaching of Pope Pius XII in the 1950s (Paris 1986, 31–32; Pius XII 1958, 395–96). It is essential to recognize that this is a moral distinction, not a medical one, and it relies on theological and philosophical understandings of the meaning of human life of which the practical implications, if not the theological bases, have largely been accepted. It is mostly a question of human benefit versus human burden.

There is no need here to go into detail about the history of the distinction. It is important to note, however, that there have been two different approaches among the moralists who have proposed it (Shannon and Walter 1988, 638). The more restrictive approach looked only to the burdens of the treatment itself. A treatment was said to be extraordinary if it was painful, caused great hardship, or was expensive. But the likely outcome, that is, the state of the patient after treatment, was not taken into consideration. The other approach, most often used today, weighs both the burdens and benefits of treatment. Here, even if the treatment itself may be inexpensive and not cause any great discomfort, it is extraordinary and therefore optional if the benefits it promises are slight or nonexistent when seen in the context of the patient's overall condition. This second approach is the one used by Gerald Kelly, arguably the most important Catholic medical ethicist prior to the Second Vatican Council of 1962–65 (Kelly 1958, 129). His definition of extraordinary means, quoted by others (McFadden 1961, 227), is given clear approval in the Declaration on Euthanasia, an official document issued by the Vatican in 1980. The declaration states that "a correct judgment can be made regarding means, if the type of treatment, its degree of difficulty and danger, its expense, and the possibility of applying it are weighed against the results that can be expected, all this in the light of the sick person's condition and resources of body and spirit" (Congregation for the Doctrine of the Faith 1998, 653). Precisely. The latest edition of the *Ethical and Religious Directives for Catholic Health Care Services* quotes this as its source in adopting the same approach (National Conference of Catholic Bishops 1995, Dirs. 56, 57). The catechism of the Catholic Church says in a similar vein, "Discontinuing medical procedures that are burdensome, dangerous, extraordinary, or disproportionate to the expected outcome can be legitimate" (*Catechism* 1994, 2278, 549).

VITALISM

The distinction between morally ordinary and morally extraordinary means of preserving life proposes a reasonable middle ground between vitalism and subjectivism, two extreme positions that are sometimes advocated. The first of these, an absolute vitalism, permits no cessation of efforts to prolong life. This position claims that life itself is the greatest possible value and it should be sustained at all costs.

A nurse once told me that she finally refused a physician's fifty-second order for cardiopulmonary resuscitation (CPR) on the same patient within forty-eight hours. Here is vitalism in the worst possible sense of the term. Perhaps it was the doctor's orders, or perhaps a surrogate was insisting that everything be done to keep the patient alive. Many hospital professionals have encountered situations in which a dying person's relatives insist that everything be done to keep their loved one alive, perhaps out of guilt, from fear of being left alone, or from a belief that Jesus may perform a miracle. In this last case, I try to suggest, gently, that Jesus—or God—does not need ventilators and defibrillators for miracles, but I have met people who are sure they have an obligation to keep a dying loved one alive as long as possible in order to give God time. No theological explanation that God does not need more time, that the ventilator and the defibrillator have already been shown to be inadequate, and so on seems to help in these cases.

Catholic medical ethicists have never considered this kind of prolongation of dying as morally required or even as a particularly good option. Theologically, I believe that Catholics' faith in the Resurrection has a good deal to do with this. The present life is to be treasured, but it is not all there is. Biological life need not be prolonged by extraordinary means.

SUBJECTIVISM

The other extreme position is a totally lax subjectivism that permits cessation of treatment, and even active killing, based only on the subjective choice of an individual. Here the idea that human life is of intrinsic value is rejected. Life is of value only if the individual gives value to it. I am convinced that there is too much of this in the United States, too much individualism, too much insistence on absolute subjective choice. I do not mean to suggest a preference

for a totalitarian or authoritarian system in which government or-
dains our values, but we are, after all, social beings. We owe help
to others precisely because they *are* of value, even if for some reason
they have lost a sense of this themselves. And U.S. law has not
moved all the way to the subjectivist extreme. Attempted suicide,
for example, though not a crime, is still a reason for insisting on
treatment, even involuntary commitment. While this can in some
cases be ill advised, even hurtful, it is good for us to maintain the
sense that human life is valuable even if an individual rejects that
value. Human life, while not of absolute value, is always intrinsically valuable. Indeed, U.S. law recognizes that the state has an
interest in preserving life, an interest in avoiding subjectivism.

Roman Catholic tradition has rejected both vitalism and subjectivism. It has recognized both the sanctity of life (life is sacred) and
the ethical import of at least some aspects of the quality of life (life
need not be prolonged under all circumstances). That is, at some
point a lack of the ability to carry out humanly meaningful purposes, which some would term a lack of quality of life, means that
life can be let go. This does not mean, however, that a person's life
loses its worth, that it ceases to be of intrinsic value. But it does
mean that when, in an individual case, the benefits of continued
living truly are outweighed by the burdens of the kind of life that
is likely to result from life-sustaining treatment and/or by the burdens of the treatment itself, the treatment may be forgone. And
Americans, as well as American law, have come to a consensus on
this. There are times when enough is enough.

The distinction between ordinary and extraordinary means of
preserving life, as I have noted, goes back several centuries. According to this tradition, one is not obliged to preserve one's life
by using measures that are morally extraordinary. The terms "ordinary" and "extraordinary" are useful, and I am hesitant to aban-
don them even in the face of some recent criticism. Critics do have
a point, however, when they argue that these words are open to
misinterpretation if the distinction is understood as a medical one
(Congregation for the Doctrine of the Faith 1998, 653). It is, rather,

a moral distinction, and there are no simple technical or statistical criteria for determining the difference. Means that are usually thought of as medically ordinary (no longer experimental, normal hospital procedures in some cases, not requiring Institutional Review Board protocol approval) may be morally extraordinary. Thus what would be an ordinary or reasonable means when used in caring for a person whose chance of renewed health is great would become extraordinary in the care of a patient who has little or no chance of recovery.

Other terms have been suggested and are in general use, but there is no pair that exactly replaces the nuances of "ordinary" and "extraordinary." "Reasonable" and "unreasonable" work in some cases, but not in others. *Unreasonable* means that the treatment is irrational. This implies that it ought not be given, whereas *extraordinary* means that the patient may choose to reject the treatment, not that it must be rejected. The treatment is optional, not necessarily wrong. "Proportionate" and "disproportionate" suffer from the same problem, as well as from the difficulty of implying a methodology about which there is considerable disagreement. "Heroic" might work, but "nonheroic" is awkward, and these terms suffer from the same problem as do the more traditional "ordinary" and "extraordinary," because they might imply that medical criteria determine the difference.

Some wish to avoid pair terms altogether and speak only of the right of autonomy, as this is guaranteed by U.S. law. But this is to restrict the issue to the legal aspects and the ethics of the law, ignoring what the Catholic tradition has properly included and what has been important in the American consensus, the moral rightness and wrongness of the decision itself. It is wrong to forgo ordinary means of preserving our lives, and there is a strong basis for this judgment. Briefly put, the dignity of human life means that we owe it to ourselves, to others, and in a very different way to God not to reject the gift of life. Because we have responsibilities to self, to others, and to God to take basic good care of ourselves, some treatments (morally ordinary) are obligatory whereas others (morally extraordinary) are optional. This is not just a decision that we make up (posit). It is a moral decision we make on the basis of what we discover objectively in the actual clinical situation.

EXAMPLES

Some examples will help clarify my statement that the distinction between ordinary and extraordinary means is a moral, not medical, one. When I give a lecture, I often ask my listeners what they would do if, right then and there, I should happen to grab my chest, groan, and fall over on the floor. The question is usually followed by silence—until someone finally says that she or he would check for a pulse and, if there is none, start CPR. Then someone else volunteers to call 911 (or, if we are in a hospital, to call a code). These, I tell them, are ordinary means of prolonging my life. In my present physical condition, I have a moral obligation to accept this treatment, to go to the emergency room and then the cardiac care unit, to take the thrombolytic agents to dissolve the blood clots, and so on. These are likely to be of real benefit to me, and objectively, this seems to outweigh the burdens. On the other hand, if we were all to come back in fifty years for an anniversary of the lecture, and I, at a very advanced age, with a multitude of diseases and previous insults, were to fall off my stretcher, gasp, and stop breathing, it would be morally right of me to have "DNR" (do not resuscitate) written on my forehead. The treatments for the cardiac arrest would be the same as before (or even more advanced), but humanly my circumstances would have changed. What was morally ordinary treatment for a person with a good chance for recovery has become morally extraordinary for one with little chance. The (human) benefits no longer outweigh the (human) burdens.

Another example concerns the use of antibiotics for pneumonia, surely a medically ordinary treatment. Yet it may be morally extraordinary for a person dying of cancer or some other serious condition. If I have been diagnosed with terminal cancer and have a few weeks to live, I might rightly see pneumonia as "the old man's friend." Of course, the medication might be morally ordinary, too—if, for example, I still had work I needed to do, such as preparing a will.

The criteria for distinguishing between morally ordinary and morally extraordinary means of prolonging life are not clean or precise. Though the distinction is an objective one in the sense that it is based on real situations, on real conditions, real prognoses, and so on, subjective elements come into play here—not subjectivism, but subjective elements. For example, a person who truly is terrified of surgery can rightly consider that fear in determining whether or not the burdens outweigh the benefits. Here terror is a real burden.

There is, then, no moral obligation to preserve life at all costs. Many factors must be weighed in this decision: the chance of success, the degree of invasiveness, pain, and patient fear, the likely outcome, the social cost (this can be quite risky, of course, and demands caution, especially in a health care system that refuses to recognize the right of all to basic care), the needs of others, the patient's readiness for death, and the patient's likely condition after successful treatment or partial success. And a person may rightly consider financial costs among the burdens. The Catholic tradition is clear about this. The sick need not sacrifice the financial survival of their families to prolong life, certainly not when the treatment is of questionable benefit and perhaps not even when the treatment is almost surely a cure. In earlier centuries, even the sense of shame or modesty a woman might feel when being examined by a male physician was sometimes said to be sufficient reason for calling the treatment extraordinary. Of course, in those days doctors were unlikely to cure, so there was far less likelihood that the treatment would do any good. The point, however, is that the distinction, as developed in Catholic medical ethics, is a flexible one.

Drawing the Line

One can describe various treatments as though they were located along a spectrum. On one end are clearly ordinary means of prolonging life: treatments such as antibiotics for pneumonia in otherwise healthy people, appendectomies, or even behaviors such as good eating habits, sufficient exercise and sleep, and so on. Then come means that most would consider ordinary but that might be extraordinary for some conditions or for some persons. After that come morally extraordinary treatments that people would be likely to consider reasonable but not obligatory—a third round of chemotherapy, for example, that might offer a small but real hope of remission for some months. A person might choose it or reject it; it is morally optional. Then, farther along on the spectrum, there are some treatments most of us would consider not only extraordinary but also unreasonable, even silly or stupid. I put feeding tubes for the irreversibly comatose in this category; yet some people, even some Catholic bishops, claim the tubes are morally required (as they did in the case of Terri Schiavo, the Florida woman said to be in a persistent vegetative state). I will return to this in chapter 6. Finally, at the extreme end of the spectrum come those procedures that are "medically futile" in the strict sense. I will examine these in detail in chapter 8.

With the exception of this last category, medical futility, the lines between the others can not be clearly drawn. There are often conflicts among those involved—patients, families, physicians, and others—a topic to which I will return in chapters 3, 4, and 5, when I examine who has the authority to make the decision. We could, I suppose, either avoid all risk of undertreatment by imposing all possible life-extending technologies on everyone or avoid all risk of overtreatment by doing nothing for anyone seriously ill. But we cannot do both, and in any case these options are clearly unacceptable. Thus despite the difficulty of drawing precise lines, the general agreement that some treatments are morally obligatory and others morally optional remains of great significance in supporting the present consensus. If the United States were basically vitalist, our laws would doubtless require that no life-sustaining treatment ever be withheld or withdrawn. If it were completely subjectivist, our laws would put no restrictions of any kind on decision making. Yet as we will see in chapter 4, the law does restrict surrogate decision making. Thus the first pillar of support, "fuzzy" as its lines may be, is essential in the present consensus on forgoing treatment.

CONCLUSION

The distinction between ordinary and extraordinary means as developed and applied within the Catholic tradition is wide and flexible. Ordinary means, which are morally obligatory, are those that offer the patient a significant human benefit without imposing a disproportionate burden. Extraordinary means, which are optional, are those that promise little significant human benefit or those that impose burdens disproportionate to the likely benefit.

The moral obligation to which this principle speaks is, of course, that of the patient. The patient is morally obliged to use ordinary or reasonable means of preserving life and is not morally obliged to use extraordinary ones. But this clearly has implications for hospital policy and for the law. If a patient is not obliged to use every possible means of preserving life, then hospitals and health care practitioners may not impose them on patients. The fact that such a distinction had been developed within Catholic medical ethics was important in developing the consensus we have reached, however tentatively, in the United States.

—⟋ *Chapter 2* ⟍—

Killing and Allowing to Die

THE second pillar of the American consensus is based on the distinction between killing and allowing to die, a distinction that Catholic tradition, in its analysis using the principle of double effect (PDE), has provided. According to this distinction, the direct killing of an innocent person is never morally right, but allowing a person to die is sometimes morally right. Some would now question the absoluteness of this distinction; that is, some now argue that direct killing (active euthanasia or assisted suicide) may be morally right in some cases. And some wish to legalize the practice. I will turn to this question in chapter 7. But the acceptance of this basic distinction has helped form both medical practice and law in the United States.

The word *euthanasia*, which comes from the Greek and means "good death" or "dying well," generally means doing something that brings about this "good" death in a person who is hopelessly ill and/or suffering pain or other burdens from an illness. The Catholic tradition sometimes uses terms like *direct* and *indirect* or *active* and *passive* euthanasia. *Direct* and *active* mean killing and are claimed to be always wrong; *indirect* and *passive* mean allowing to die and are, therefore, sometimes right. But I am convinced that it is better to avoid confusion and use the word "euthanasia" only to refer to the actual killing of a patient.

Catholic tradition states the second pillar thus: It is always morally wrong to directly kill an innocent person, but it is sometimes morally right to allow a person to die. Two simple words here are at times overlooked: "always" and "sometimes." The norm is not that it is always wrong to kill and always right to allow to die; dismissing the norm on the basis that it is not always right to allow people to die misses the basic point. Clearly, it is sometimes wrong to allow people to die of their illnesses. If I arrive at an emergency room (ER) at a full service hospital in the United States with acute appendicitis and am denied an appendectomy because I lack insurance, and I die in the ER, the hospital has not in fact killed me. No one has shot me or injected me with a lethal dose of medication. It has (only) allowed me to die. But in doing so, it has done me a great injustice. It has also broken the law. I am convinced that a consistent understanding of the distinction between killing and allowing to die requires the insistence that some incidents of allowing to die, even though they are not killings in the strictest sense, may nonetheless be morally wrong.

FIVE TYPES OF ACTIONS

There are five different kinds of actions to be considered in a discussion of the distinction between killing and allowing to die.

Withholding Life-Sustaining Treatment

One may decide not to use certain medical means that would prolong life (not to use a ventilator for a terminally ill patient, for example, or not to resuscitate a patient who suffers from some severe illness). This withholding of treatment is not the killing of a person; it is an allowing to die. It is not always morally right, but it is sometimes, indeed it is often, morally right. If the means in question are "morally extraordinary," the act (the decision not to use the means) is generally accepted as moral.

Withdrawing Life-Sustaining Treatment

One may decide to stop the use of a means that has already been begun (to withdraw a treatment, to turn off the ventilator, to "pull the plug," to "do a terminal wean"). Catholic moral tradition considers this action the equivalent of withholding life-sustaining treatment. Morally, assuming the burdens outweigh the benefits, it is the nonuse of extraordinary means and is normal procedure in U.S. hospitals. Until the American consensus was achieved, this second kind of action was sometimes considered, from a legal standpoint, more dangerous, more open to repercussion or at least to malpractice litigation, as it is physically the actual doing of something rather than the simple nondoing of it. But recent court decisions, especially the Supreme Court decisions in the *Cruzan* case (*Cruzan v. Director*, 1990) and on physician-assisted suicide (*Vacco v. Quill*, 1997; *Washington v. Glucksberg*, 1997), have made it clear that withdrawing treatment is legally the equivalent of withholding it.

Thus it can now be stated that if it is morally right and legal to withhold treatment X in circumstances ABC, then it is morally right and legal to withdraw treatment X in the same circumstances. The circumstances may change, of course, as when patients or surrogates state that they would have withheld treatment but are now unwilling to withdraw it. But that is a question of who decides. There is no ethical or legal difference between withholding and withdrawing.

This understanding is important for a number of reasons. The most obvious is that otherwise we would be forced to maintain useless and unwanted treatment—and forced to use scarce resources in doing so. But there is a danger of undertreatment as well. If patients and their families were to fear that certain procedures, such as placing a patient on a ventilator, could never be reversed, they might be overly hesitant to authorize them in the first place. I have been involved in a number of cases in which families needed assurance that a ventilator was not a sentence to permanent medical imprisonment. They may have remembered hearing of instances in which families were denied permission to turn them off even when they were doing no human good. Sometimes early discussion with patients and their families can result in withholding unwanted and nonbeneficial treatment so that the emotionally more difficult later decision to withdraw is not necessary. In many cases, however, this is not possible because the prognosis is not yet clear. Families need to be assured that, after a time-limited trial, medical procedures that turn out to be ineffective can be discontinued. Additionally, if withdrawal of treatment is not allowed, people might insist in their advance directives that they never want certain procedures (intubation seems the most common fear) regardless of the outcome. And ER physicians might be overly hesitant to begin emergency care, fearing that later diagnostic tests could show such treatments to be unwarranted. The moral and legal identity of withholding and withdrawing, which has its origins in Catholic ethics, is thus essential to good ethics, good law, and good medicine.

Though moralists of earlier times often used the terms "negative euthanasia" or "passive euthanasia" (or, more technically within Roman Catholic moral theology, "indirect euthanasia") to refer to either withholding or withdrawing treatment, it seems far better, as I have already noted, not to use the word "euthanasia" to apply to either of them. It is less confusing if we reserve this word for the actual killing of patients. Neither withholding nor withdrawing medical treatments are acts of killing. Rather, they allow the patient to die of the underlying condition. They are not always morally right. But "allowing to die" is morally right when it is the forgoing of morally extraordinary treatment. Withholding and withdrawing may feel different, but ethically and legally there is no reason to distinguish them.

Pain Relief that Hastens (Co-Causes) Death

One may take positive means aimed at relieving the patient's suffering, but not directly intended to cause death, even though the drug administered may indeed "co-cause," or hasten, death. For example, in some rare cases patients build up such a tolerance to a drug that the dose needed to eliminate pain will suppress respiration and thus be a causal factor in their death, but it is still morally right and legal to use that needed dosage. It is certainly a moral act to relieve pain, and this sort of medication cannot be considered ethically wrong, as long as consideration is given to the patient's wishes. The Catholic tradition tends to call this third kind of action *indirect killing*. To understand this, it is necessary to introduce the principle of double effect. From a theoretical perspective, there are a number of serious problems with the PDE, but those problems do not directly affect its application to the issue of pain relief and so we can be brief.

The principle of double effect claims to answer the following question: Is it right to perform an action from which two or more effects result, some of which are good and may rightly be intended and some of which are bad and may not rightly be intended? The principle proposes that an action with both good and bad effects is right if and only if all four of the following conditions are met: (1) the act-in-itself must not be morally wrong, (2) the bad effect must not cause the good effect, (3) the agent must not intend the bad effect, and (4) the bad effect must not outweigh the good effect.

The use of medication to relieve pain in a dying patient even at the foreseen risk of hastening death meets the requirements of the PDE. Indeed, it is sometimes called *double-effect euthanasia*, a term that is better not used because of the confusion it causes. Pain relief that hastens death meets the first condition of the PDE because the act itself is not a killing but an administration of medication that relieves pain. It meets the second because the bad effect, death, is not caused by the good effect, pain relief. Rather, the medication causes both with equal causal immediacy. Third, the intention of the agent is not that the patient be dead but that the patient be free of pain. And fourth, in the case of a dying patient, the bad effect, a slightly earlier death, is outweighed by the good effect, the relief of pain. Thus this action, like the first two, may well be morally right according to Catholic moral tradition. And in the U.S. legal and ethical consensus, the same judgment is made.

This means that it is always medically possible, and, assuming the proper decision maker agrees, it is always morally right and always legal to *eliminate* physical pain in the imminently dying patient. It is extremely important to stress this, because some claim that there are exceptions, that is, that there are cases in which complete pain relief is not possible even for an imminently dying person. But if we look more closely at the reasons for this claim, we find that none of them are valid.

The three most commonly cited arguments for why elimination of pain in a dying patient is not always possible are as follows. First, there is fear of addiction. I am glad to say that in the past few years, whenever I have mentioned this, listeners have laughed. And it is indeed laughable. Addiction is certainly an important problem for those whose unwarranted use of drugs causes harm to their lives and the lives of others. Heroin, cocaine, alcohol, nicotine, and other agents, including drugs such as morphine used by doctors for pain relief, can cause great damage when they are improperly used. For an imminently dying patient, however, pain medication is not addictive in this sense. The term *addiction* indicates both a description of a physical condition (withdrawal causes physical symptoms) and a social condition. In this latter sense, addiction is a social construct. It connotes crime, violence, the need for rehabilitation, and so on. None of these are present in the imminently dying patient. A person dying of cancer on a morphine drip is unlikely to go out and rob a liquor store for a fix. Recent medical literature has claimed that even physical addiction is very rare in people who need opiates for pain relief. Even the nondying person is unlikely to become physically addicted to a drug given for relief of pain. Usually, when the source of the pain is ended, the drugs are ended, too, without symptoms of withdrawal. In any case, even if there is some physical addiction, it is irrelevant in the case of dying patients who need pain relief as they die.

The second reason sometimes given for why it may be impossible to eliminate pain in some dying patients is that an increase in the drug will cause death. But we have just seen why this is not a problem. As long as the amount of drug given is what is needed to relieve pain, and as long as no one intends the patient's death, the drug increase is morally right and legal. Concerning the amount of drug given and the way it is administered, physicians need simply to follow the standard range suggested for this patient's condition in these circumstances. The standard of medical care clearly permits using enough drug to eliminate pain in these patients. Doctors need to be sure they do not give an amount so clearly beyond what is needed that the only reason for doing so would be to kill the patient. And, especially in the case of a "terminal wean" (withdrawal of a ventilator even though the doctors know the patient will not be able to breathe unassisted—I dislike this phrase, but I fear we are stuck with it), physicians should make sure they avoid using phrases such as "Let's give the patient enough morphine to prevent any attempt at breathing." This can be used as legal evidence that the doctor indeed intended to kill the patient.

In such cases, questions regarding the intention of the physician or the family may arise, but they are easily resolved. It is understandable and even praiseworthy that the family and the doctor may see the earlier death, if it occurs, as a blessing. They may be glad that the patient's long illness and dying process are over. The family may even be relieved to get back to their lives and their families. None of this means they "intended" the patient's death in the sense meant by the Catholic tradition or by U.S. law. But families may feel guilty about withholding or withdrawing treatment or about pain relief when this may hasten death. Because they say things such as "Let him die a natural death," "Let him die with dignity," "Let him be at peace with God," or "His death will be a blessing," they may worry that they somehow intend their loved one's death. There is a simple way to alleviate such anxiety, and it is by asking them if they would want their loved one with them if a cure were possible. Of course they say yes. This means they do not intend death; they do not want their loved one dead. Thus, the question to ask in deciding whether or not family members intend death is, If there were an alternative (a cure) that would cause the good effect (freedom from the dying process) and not cause the bad effect (death), would you choose that alternative? Families inevitably say yes. And this relieves them from at least some of the worry that so often accompanies this kind of decision.

The third reason given for why it is sometimes not possible to alleviate a dying patient's pain is that the amount of drug needed to do so will render the person unconscious as he or she dies. This is sometimes called *terminal sedation*, another term I do not like because it can easily be taken to mean active euthanasia. I prefer the term *palliative sedation*, as suggested by James Walter (2002, 6). This is indeed a case where pain relief "fails," but only insofar as it fails to do what is the ideal. It fails to eliminate the pain while leaving the person alert and capable of interaction. But surely this is no reason to reject pain relief in the dying patient if the patient or surrogate asks for it. If the patient decides it is better to stop the pain than to be conscious and in constant agony, surely that wish must be followed. And there is general agreement that surrogates may not legally or morally reject pain medication for dying people.

There are cases, of course, in which dying people themselves choose to suffer pain rather than lose their capacity to complete tasks they wish to do before dying. In these cases, the wishes of competent people should be followed. Cases in which people have written in their advance treatment directives that they refuse pain relief (perhaps out of guilt or fear of God) are extremely rare, and I must admit that I would try to override such directives for now-incompetent patients, following a surrogate's decision to relieve pain or seeking legal relief from the directive if necessary.

However, although it is right and legal to eliminate physical pain, the same does not necessarily apply to other kinds of human suffering. James Walter makes a helpful distinction between "neurophysiological suffering" and what he calls "agent narrative suffering" (Walter 2002, 6). The former is what we usually mean by *pain* and includes the kind of physiological distress that comes from the experienced inability to breathe. This pain can and ought to be eliminated. But the latter, the other kind of human suffering—

worries about dying, guilt for past sins, concern for family, a sense of hopelessness—is sometimes a human reality that people have to deal with. I do not mean that these kinds of sufferings should be ignored by physicians and others involved with the dying patient. Dying people often reach out to others for conversation, therapy, prayer, and other kinds of interaction. And when these anxieties threaten to overwhelm, there is nothing that forbids alleviating them by medication. But often they call more for compassion and communication than for sedation. Such anxieties are, in any case, not the physical pain that can be eliminated.

(Physician)-Assisted Suicide

One may act in conjunction with the patient by assisting him or her in active euthanasia. The patient wishes to die, makes this known to the health care practitioner—asking the practitioner to provide the necessary means—and the patient actually consumes the drug or initiates the suicide. This is assisted suicide in the strict sense. It is a direct self-killing. In the Catholic tradition (and until recently in the American moral consensus) it is judged to be wrong. In addition, assisting in suicide is illegal in most, though not in all, U.S. jurisdictions. The most obvious exception is Oregon.

(Active) Euthanasia

The health care practitioner may take action that directly causes the patient's death. This, like assisted suicide, is referred to as *positive euthanasia, active euthanasia,* or, within the Catholic tradition, *direct euthanasia.* It is a direct killing according to the principle of double effect and is considered first-degree murder in all jurisdictions. To my knowledge, however, until the conviction of Jack Kevorkian in Michigan, no physician had been convicted of the crime of killing a dying patient, though family members have been. I will return to the question of physician-assisted suicide and euthanasia in chapter 7.

—✂ *Chapter 3* ✂—

Decisions by Competent Patients

I N chapters 1 and 2 I discussed the first two pillars that support the present American consensus on forgoing treatment, the two that are based in Catholic medical ethics. The third pillar has its basis in law and derives from the legal concept of the right to privacy, autonomy, and liberty. This has been interpreted to mean that patients capable of making decisions of this type may refuse treatment even against the advice of their physicians. The patient has the right of autonomy to choose and of privacy to be left alone. The Supreme Court's June 1990 *Cruzan* decision, which relied on common-law liberties, established as the law of the land the right of competent patients to refuse treatment (*Cruzan v. Director*, 1990). Similarly, the courts in most cases have decided that patients not capable of making decisions may also refuse treatment through surrogate decision makers.

The precise relationship between this third pillar (the right of privacy, autonomy, and liberty) and the first pillar (the difference between mandatory and optional treatment) is not yet theoretically clear, though in most jurisdictions the practical judgments rendered have led to consistent outcomes. Not theoretically clear is the question of what legal implications follow from the distinction between reasonable and unreasonable (or ordinary and extraordinary) treatment. Though we cannot here explore the complex theoretical issues, we will look closely at their practical implications. We have seen that the moral obligation to use reasonable or morally ordinary means to preserve life falls primarily on the patient. But what if a patient deemed capable of making such decisions chooses to forgo a means of treatment that, in any reasonable judgment, is "ordinary," beneficial, inexpensive, and of little burden? I go to the hospital with a pain that is diagnosed as acute appendicitis, but, after admission, I refuse permission for surgery. What moral obligation does this bring to the health care institution and its practitioners? Should this have any bearing on the courts' decisions or on the legality of forgoing treatment?

In practical terms, courts have tended to resolve such questions by upholding the right of patients to refuse for themselves with little or no insistence on the distinction between reasonable and unreasonable treatments. Of course, the fact that a person refuses a treatment that seems reasonable might be an indication that the person lacks the capacity to decide. But it might not be, as, for example, in the case of a person who refuses treatment for religious reasons. Treatment generally considered reasonable or ordinary might be judged unreasonable, even repugnant, by such a patient. The right of autonomy and privacy has prevailed in those cases in which the patient is capable of deciding.

Legal Basis

There are three sources of U.S. law. First, there is statutory law, that is, laws passed by legislatures on the federal, state, and sometimes local level. Second, there is the U.S. Constitution and interpretations of that document in state courts, federal courts, and, ultimately, the U.S. Supreme Court. Third, there is common law, which is the totality of court cases that have resolved certain issues and become a kind of unwritten and universally accepted complex of laws and codes of conduct. Because some common law was adapted from English law before the American Revolution, we sometimes refer to *Anglo-Saxon common law.*

Legal scholars have looked at this third pillar and have identified several possible sources for the generally accepted legal conclusion that patients have the authority to decide about treatment. Some suggest that it comes from the right to privacy or autonomy found in the Constitution. Others argue that a better source is the common-law liberty to refuse unwanted treatment, which is part of the common-law liberty to refuse unwanted touching. This source is the clearest, the oldest, and the least controversial basis for the right to refuse treatment. The right to privacy has been found in the Constitution only recently (applied in the context of abortion and birth control, controversial issues in their own right).[1] All agree that no one has an absolute right to privacy or autonomy, only a few claim that the state has no right to tax us, and the Constitution gives us only a freedom from unreasonable search and seizure, not from all search and seizure.

The common-law basis does not suffer as much from controversy or ambiguity of this kind. No one may touch me without my consent. Admittedly, there are times when I must give my consent, as to customs officials who search my person or police officers who arrest me, but these are rare exceptions and they are rather clear. The common-law liberty to refuse unwanted touching is really common sense. States do not need statutes that forbid one person from hitting or beating another, or statutes that forbid unwanted sexual touching. It is simply clear that people have the right to refuse such attacks. And the same applies to unwanted medical treatment. Individuals have the right to decline such interventions.

THE ACE OF TRUMP

The right of refusal by competent patients is the only ace of trump in the context of legal authority to refuse treatment. Although "competent" is not really the right word here, since it refers technically to a court decision, "decision-making capable" is so awkward that "competent" has generally replaced it. If a person who is clearly capable of making the decision refuses treatment, the physician may not treat. Treating in this case is criminal assault and battery. Even the threat to treat is assault. If a competent patient says, "I do not want any more chemotherapy" and the doctor replies, "You're going to get it anyway, if I have to hold you down and make you take it," that physician has already criminally assaulted the patient, even if he has no intention of following through on the threat and says it just to get the patient to acquiesce. And if nurses, following the physician's orders, begin to restrain the patient, both they and the doctor have assaulted and battered the patient.

EXCEPTIONS THAT SELDOM TRUMP THE ACE OF TRUMP

Theoretically there are two exceptions in law to the right of competent persons to refuse treatment: the exception sometimes made for pregnant women and the exception sometimes made for parents, usually mothers, of small children. But the first of these hardly ever occurs, and the second, though courts used to impose it on occasion, has to my knowledge not been imposed in recent U.S. court decisions.

Pregnant Women

Some courts and some state laws have made an exception for a pregnant woman, but this issue is very controversial, and courts often allow both the woman and fetus to die if the woman refuses treatment (Meisel 1989, 110–12; 1995, 1:645–53; 2003, 258). Some advance directive statutes, such as Pennsylvania's Advance Directive for Health Care Act, include an exception for a woman whose fetus might be brought to the stage of viability. But advance directive acts do not apply to presently competent patients, so they do not affect the contemporaneous decision of a competent woman. And, of course, the woman may choose an abortion, which would render the whole issue moot. Indeed, the exception clause for pregnant women clearly stands in tension with the abortion decisions in *Roe v. Wade* (1973) and *Doe v. Bolton* (1973). It is inconsistent on the one hand to allow abortions at the pure choice of the woman and on the other to insist that she cannot refuse life-sustaining treatment for herself if she is pregnant and the fetus can be saved. The right to refuse treatment is far better based in ethics and in law than is the right to abort.

Parents of Small Children

In the past, courts have sometimes required reasonable ("ordinary") treatment to save the lives of parents whose children would otherwise be left orphans, but they have recently stopped doing this (Meisel 1989, 102–3; 1995, 1:516–24; 2003, 229). The exception was more often imposed on mothers than on fathers and therefore has been perceived as sexist. In addition, U.S. law has been moving in the direction of the defense of individual rights and of each person's right to control his or her body regardless of other factors. Thus, parents are usually now given the same right as nonparents to refuse life-sustaining treatment, even if that treatment seems medically indicated or morally ordinary.

STILL THE ACE OF TRUMP

The distinction between kinds of treatment has generally not been a major factor in the right of a competent person to refuse treatment. Even though we might wish to say that we have a *moral* obligation to take reasonable care of ourselves, to use morally ordinary means to preserve our lives, the *law* does not recognize this as an obligation for competent persons. If a person capable of making this kind of decision decides to refuse life-sustaining treatment, that decision stands.

Illustrative Case

I come to the hospital's emergency room with pain in my lower abdomen, which is quickly diagnosed as acute appendicitis. I am otherwise healthy. The doctor tells me I need an appendectomy. I say, "No! Take anything else out, but not my appendix." The doctor tells me that appendectomies are common and without one I will almost certainly die. I reply, "I'm terribly sorry, but I belong to the Anti-Appendectomy Sect of the Old Irish Catholic Church. We believe that the appendix is where God keeps our souls. If you take it out, I can never get to heaven to meet St. Patrick." My doctor, if he knows me well, might say that's the silliest thing he's ever heard.

Then I ask the doctor, "Do you believe in God?" He tells me yes, that he's even Catholic, but he's never heard of this Old Irish thing. I ask, "Does God act stupidly?" The doctor's answer: "No, of course not." I then ask what the appendix is for, and the doctor admits to having no idea. I tell him that we Old Irish know what it's for, since St. Patrick left a hidden message for us telling us that our souls are in our appendices and we should never let go of them. I take out my Old Irish wallet card that reads "In an emergency, call an Old Irish priest, but never ever take out my appendix." The doctor, to make sure this is a real church, calls the number on the card, and it is answered by the headquarters of the Old Irish Anti-Appendectomy Church. They confirm this, even providing their tax exemption number, which the doctor confirms with the IRS. My doctor tries once more: "Once your appendix ruptures, your soul gets loose anyhow." I say that's irrelevant, because God will keep my soul in a small part of my appendix that will not rupture.

I have raised this seemingly silly case as a way of making it clear that one can be a competent person holding to a consistent belief that may well risk his or her life. If I tell my doctor that I will accept the use of antibiotics and other treatments, but not an appendectomy, that is that. If the surgery is done despite my refusal, it is criminal assault and battery. There is no possible reason to think that I am deluded by sepsis (I have the card and the phone number; my belief is not new). There is no internal inconsistency in my belief; I have thought it out well. I am aware of my condition as it now is. I am aware that I may well die because of my refusal. I am aware that the operation itself is common and will doubtless save my life. I still refuse. Game over. Ace of trump wins. Supreme Court decisions have established this as the law of the land.

Persuasion

None of this means that health care professionals are reduced to silence when a patient refuses a treatment that will offer clear benefit, a treatment that will "fix" the problem. They are the experts in medicine, and they should try to convince patients to accept beneficial treatments. They serve life when medicine truly saves lives, and I believe it is correct to "err on the side of life," as long as this often-used phrase is properly interpreted and applied. When it is clear that life cannot be served, that is, when the proposed treatment is morally extraordinary, to err on its side is wrongheaded at best and possibly immoral and illegal. But health care professionals ought to try to persuade patients to accept treatments with a reasonable chance of success. I do not accept the idea that physicians are merely "providers" of procedures to "consumers" who choose them and pay for them. The relationship is much more than that. It includes trust and is a covenant between people seeking a common goal (May 1983). Health professionals are, I think, right to try to persuade their patients to do what is in the patients' best interests. They rightly tell patients to stop smoking, to change diet, to use this or that medicine. They rightly argue and try to convince, just as the fictional doctor did in the strange appendix case above. But the final decision rests with the competent patient.

Demand for Treatment Is Not an Ace of Trump

Competent patients do not have a legal right to demand treatment. Though the contemporaneous decision of a competent person to refuse treatment is legally definitive (with the two possible but unlikely exceptions I have noted), the same cannot be said for the decision to request a treatment. Persons cannot ask for treatments that are contrary to the standards of medical care. They cannot pick and choose which treatments they want. They cannot demand treatment A and reject B if B is necessary for A to work. I will return to this point in chapter 8.

Waiver of Decision-Making Authority by Competent Patients

The fact that competent patients have the legal right to decide about their treatment, to accept or reject the treatment the physician recommends, does not mean that they need to exercise that right by making decisions themselves. They can and sometimes do delegate that authority to someone else. This is most likely to happen when patients feel that someone else, usually a close family member, will understand the medical complexities better than they could themselves. In some cases this may indicate that the patient is really not fully able to make these decisions, but in other cases it is more a matter of preference.

Some of the most difficult cases involve patients from cultures in which custom dictates that other family members, often the oldest male, make medical decisions. Here it is not enough to know that, for example, the patient wants her son to decide. Doctors, or social workers or chaplains, should try to gently find out why this is the patient's wish. Perhaps she does not agree with the custom but is being forced to comply. Or perhaps the custom itself is so unjust that the physician may decide not to honor it. Insoo Hyun argues that "to be autonomous, a person must also have authentic moral values. She must act on her own values, not on values that were improperly impressed upon her" (Hyun 2002, 14). Yet it is hard to know exactly what "improperly impressed" means. These are difficult cases, and there is no single norm for solving them. In any case, I do not agree that a physician should simply accept the family's word that they, not the patient, should be informed and should give consent. At the very least, such patients must be informed that in the United States it is the law that they be allowed to make their own decisions if they wish to do so. Then they should be asked if they want to keep or waive their right to do this.

What Is Competence?

The issue of determining capacity to make decisions of this kind is so complex that I will not attempt here to go into detail (see Grisso and Applebaum 1998). The basic idea is that people have the right to give free and informed consent to medical treatment or to freely and understandingly refuse that consent. To do this, they need to have the capacity to choose freely and to understand what is being asked of them. The factors that might reduce or eliminate freedom and understanding are so many and so controversial that no exhaustive treatment is possible. Indeed, if *free and informed consent* is taken to mean "free from all outside influence whatsoever and informed at the level of medical experts," then true consent is seldom if ever possible. But such a definition is wrong. The human person is not an isolated individual, free from all social influence and interaction. Perfectly competent patients will quite rightly take into account the wishes of their families and others who may be influencing their decisions, and such influence does not mean that the consent is not free.

Some general criteria are used to determine if a patient has decision-making capacity. I included many of them in the antiappendectomist case. The patient must be free from all openly coercive influence. If a physician suspects such influence may be present, the patient should be questioned alone. The patient must be able to understand in basic human terms the diagnosis and prognosis and the risks and benefits of the treatment, as well as any reasonable alternative approaches. The physician is legally required to give whatever information the patient reasonably needs to make an informed judgment (Meisel 1989, 28–29; 1995, 1:95–97). Heather Gert suggests that it is better to give more than this, to give enough so that the patient "will not be surprised by whatever happens—unless the physician is also surprised" (Gert 2002, 23). And the physician should supply information in language the patient can understand. I have taken part in many consultations in which this was the key issue. Patients (or, if the patient is not competent, surrogate decision makers) are all too often given medical jargon, and in the frequently overwhelming context of the modern hospital, they may well nod and say they understand. But how is a patient or a family to know that a *total bilateral occipital infarct* means permanent blindness unless the doctor takes the time to say that? The patient should be able to answer the doctor's well-worded questions: "Do you understand that you will be blind?" and "What will that mean for you?"

The competent patient's decisions will exhibit consistency. This means two things. First, the decisions reached on Monday should not differ substantially from those reached on Wednesday unless the patient's condition has changed or unless she is able to articulate why she has changed her mind. Second, the decisions reached should be consistent with the patient's own articulated values. If a patient says that he wants to be allowed to die in peace and then insists on CPR after cardiac arrest, it may be that he does not understand what CPR is, in which case the doctor should tell him, or it may be that he is not able to understand. Usually conversation will disclose which is the case. In any case, competent patients will be able to articulate to some degree a consistent sense of what their goals are, as well as to understand how suggested treatments would affect those goals.

It is important to note that competence in this sense is relative to the kind of decision that is to be made. Decision-making capacity should be seen more as a sliding scale than as an either/or judgment. Patients who cannot balance their checkbooks or do their own taxes may be perfectly able to understand their diagnosis and prognosis and the treatment options available to them. On the other hand, deciding about life-sustaining treatment requires more capacity than deciding what to order for supper. And it is often the case that patients are more capable at certain times of the day than at others, or more capable just before or just after a medication is administered. Effort needs to be taken to accommodate these differences.

I worry more about capacity in patients who reject ordinary means of getting better than in those who reject extraordinary means. The decision to reject a truly beneficial treatment is simply less "reasonable," as most "reasonable people" would accept this kind of treatment. I do not mean by this that the values of the physician, or even that of reasonable people, should trump the values of patients. I hope that the anti-appendectomist case has made that clear. But decisions to reject clearly beneficial treatments call for greater attention to patient capacity than do decisions to accept such treatments.

In most cases it is easy to tell whether a patient is competent to make treatment decisions. There is no legal requirement that a neurologist or psychiatrist be consulted; the attending physician usually knows if the patient is competent (Meisel 1989, 211–13; 1995, 1:174–79). But in some cases a psychological or neurological consultation may help. Experience tells us, however, that these consultations are far more helpful when the consulting specialists are made aware of the context rather than simply called to do a general work-up. The fact that a patient is "oriented times three" (able to give his or her name, location, and the date) is seldom very helpful.

One issue that often arises is the problem of depression.[2] Sometimes a clinical depression means that a patient lacks capacity to decide about treatment. But sadness and hopelessness are not the same as clinical depression, and not all depressions impede this kind of decision-making capacity, as we are starting to learn. Feeling hopeless is not at all irrational when faced with a terminal diagnosis. We need to understand this and not assume that depressed patients cannot make a free and informed consent about treatment (Grisso and Applebaum 1998, 9, 57).

A second question now being raised more formally is that of competence in adolescents. State laws are often of little help here, in that they simply determine an age of majority—often eighteen—and then make some statutory exceptions to it for so-called emancipated minors. These exceptions may include married teenagers, military personnel, or girls seeking abortions or contraceptives. Legal investigations by Rhonda Gay Hartman have disclosed that there is significant legal precedent for heeding the wishes of adolescents (Hartman 2000, 2001). The general principle is in any case clear, at least in theory. The decision to forgo treatment made by a person capable of making it must be followed. The question thus is whether or not a particular adolescent is capable of making this kind of decision. In many cases adolescents are quite capable of doing this. All the same restrictions and concerns that I have described as applying to adults apply also, of course, to adolescents. And it should be noted that adolescents' capacity for competence varies widely according to age and experience; twelve-year-olds and seventeen-year-olds have very different capacities. Still, I do not think clear lines can be drawn, and I cannot see any reason for keeping adolescents out of the conversation.

Catholic Hospitals and Competent Patients Rejecting Ordinary Means

I began this chapter by noting that the relationship between the first pillar (ordinary and extraordinary means) and the third pillar (the legal right of a patient to refuse treatment) is not theoretically clear. Yet it has become clear in practice, at least as regards patients with decision-making capacity. They may legally reject any and all treatment, even if to most of us that treatment would appear morally ordinary. What is the ethical obligation of Catholic hospitals when faced with a decision by a capable patient to refuse morally ordinary treatment? What should a Catholic hospital do if the anti-appendectomist arrives at its ER? Or what should it do if a Jehovah's Witness comes with an easily treatable but potentially fatal loss of blood?

The *Ethical and Religious Directives*, a set of policies for Catholic health care institutions issued by the American Catholic Bishops, are not particularly helpful here. Directive 59, which concerns the decision of a competent patient to forgo life-sustaining treatment, states: "The free and informed judgment made by a competent adult patient concerning the use or withdrawal of life-sustaining procedures should always be respected and normally complied with, unless it is contrary to Catholic moral teaching" (United States Conference of Catholic Bishops 2001, Dir. 59). The rejection of morally ordinary treatment is, presumably, "contrary to Catholic moral teaching," but U.S. law is quite clear that judgments of competent adults to refuse treatment must always be complied with, whether or not they are in keeping with Catholic moral teaching. Are Catholic hospitals obliged to violate the law against assault and battery by forcing life-sustaining procedures on competent patients?

Perhaps this question can be answered by arguing that for these patients the treatments are morally extraordinary—the ordinary-extraordinary distinction, as we have seen, does admit of a good deal of subjective variation—but in some cases this approach gives a more relativist twist to that distinction than I think it is good for it to bear. For example, do we want to say that appendectomies for acute appendicitis in otherwise healthy individuals become morally extraordinary when the sick person is an anti-appendectomist? If we say this, it becomes morally right for the anti-appendectomist to reject surgery. Or we might prefer to say that the treatment is objectively morally ordinary, so that although the patient's rejection is ethically wrong, he is not personally blameworthy (or guilty of sinning) because he does not understand, as a result of his religious beliefs, his obligation to have the appendectomy. Saying that the treatment is for him morally ordinary is the more irenic way of approaching this—we might well do that for the Jehovah's Witness who refuses blood—yet it is puzzling to call this treatment "morally extraordinary" while maintaining that this distinction is basically an objective one, as I think we have to do.[3]

In any case, it is clear that Catholic hospitals are not expected to assault their patients. Unlike certain procedures that Catholic hospitals are told to avoid (direct abortion or direct sterilization, for example), this would be a case of requiring them to violate the basic right of a person not to be treated against his or her will. Catholic hospitals could ask competent patients who refuse morally ordinary means to seek help elsewhere, but surely this would not be a common practice.

Is the Law Morally Right?

We have seen that there is an ethical obligation to use ordinary means of treatment, and we have found that the law grants competent patients the right to refuse this very treatment. What are we to say about the ethical rightness or wrongness of the law here? Is the law contrary to Catholic ethics? Is it contrary to bioethics in general? Ought we try to change it so that competent patients are legally obliged to do what they are ethically obliged to do: take decent care of themselves?

It is helpful in this context to distinguish three levels of judgment: (1) the moral rightness or wrongness of the action (the decision to forgo ordinary treatment), (2) the legal status of the action, and (3) the moral rightness and wrongness of the law establishing the legal status. In the case in which I choose to reject a morally ordinary means of preserving my life, the answer to (1) is that I act wrongly, though I may or may not be morally blameworthy in doing so—that depends on subjective factors such as knowledge and consent. The answer to (2) is that the law says no one can force me to have the treatment. And the answer to (3) is, in my judgment, that the law upholding the right of competent patients to refuse treatment is a morally right, a just, law.

I am not sure I can prove this claim. I take seriously the state's interest in preserving life. Yet I worry about the state imposing its power against the free decisions of clearly competent people concerning their own health and the treatment they do or do not want. There is something wholesome about the tendency in U.S. law not to intervene in personal decisions. I believe that in the final analysis we are, when considering the contemporaneous decision of a competent person, better off running the risk of a bad decision than running the risk of governmental interference. As we have seen, the distinction between ordinary and extraordinary, while basically an objective one, includes subjective elements. When competent patients decide for themselves, they are better able than others to take account of these elements. It would be difficult for the courts or other outsiders to determine which treatments should be imposed and which should not. But this difficulty, great as it is, cannot excuse the law from trying to make similar judgments when surrogates decide to forgo treatment for incompetent patients (I will turn to this complex question in the next chapter). When surrogates decide, the state simply must require that certain standards be followed.

Conclusion

The right of a patient capable of making free and informed consent to refuse any and all medical treatment is firmly established in U.S. law. The decision of a competent patient to refuse treatment is the "ace of trump" or the "gold standard" as far as the law is concerned. We can now turn to more complicated matters. What happens when we cannot get the contemporaneous decision of a competent person? Here we will see that although the law tries to get as close as it can to the gold standard, this sometimes leads to considerable difficulties.

Notes

1. The right to privacy was first articulated by the Supreme Court in *Griswold v. Connecticut* (1965), the case that struck down a statute forbidding contraception, and was repeated in *Roe v. Wade* (1973), the decision legalizing abortion, then in *In re Quinlan* (1976), and often since then. An excellent review of this is found in a paper by David S. Pollock and Todd M. Begg (1990). The *Cruzan* decision (1990) did indeed base itself on this sort of liberty rather than on the right to privacy, and in this the decision was correct. The liberty was claimed on the basis of the Fourteenth Amendment.

2. The ethical issues pertaining to mental health are many and complex. Though much of what is treated in this book can be applied to mental health care, I have not attempted to investigate those issues in detail. For one approach to a Catholic ethic of mental health care, see Ashley and O'Rourke 1997, 355–94. For an investigation of mental health issues in the context of managed care, see Nelson 2003.

3. For a Catholic defense of the right of Jehovah's Witnesses to refuse blood, see Devine 1989.

—◌ৎ *Chapter 4* ৎ◌—

Decisions for Incompetent Patients

THUS far in my discussion of the third pillar of the American consensus, I have focused on the decisions of competent patients, cases in which the problems are not as difficult as those concerning incompetent patients. As we have seen, the "gold standard" or the "ace of trump" in these matters is the decision of a competent patient. But when a patient is not able to make decisions, this ace of trump is not possible. In such cases, U.S. law, with its emphasis on individual autonomy, tries to get as close as it can to the gold standard.

The question is: How can we try to follow the wishes of a person who cannot now tell us what he or she wants? The brief answer is that treatment decisions will be made by a surrogate, a substitute decision maker for the patient. Surrogate decision makers, however, do not have the same total authority as the competent person. There is only one ace of trump. Surrogates are legally and ethically held to certain standards.

A good, basic rule to follow when faced with surrogate decision making is this: Ordinarily, surrogates may not choose to forgo (withhold or withdraw) treatment when that treatment is in the objective best interests of the patient. There may be an exception to this, such as when an advance directive specifically rejects a treatment. But even here we need to be very careful before we reject a treatment that has a good chance of success. Advance directives, as we shall see in the next chapter, always require interpretation. In my experience, people almost never mean to reject truly beneficial treatment in their advance directives. They may say they never want CPR after their heart stops, but they do not mean they would reject CPR if they were electrocuted and could recover. They may say they never want a ventilator, but they mean they would not want to be tethered to it if they have little or no hope of ever getting off; they would not reject it for a few days in, for example, an acute case of pneumonia that would probably respond to antibiotics. And in the rare cases in which people really do mean to reject what most of us think of as morally ordinary or reasonable treatment, it is usually convincingly clear why they do so, as, for example, when a Jehovah's Witness writes an advance directive rejecting blood transfusion.

This position is not idiosyncratic. In *Principles of Biomedical Ethics*, Beauchamp and Childress write:

> We believe the best interests standard . . . can in some circumstances validly override advance directives executed by autonomous patients who have now become incompetent, refusals by minors, and refusals by other incompetent patients. This overriding can occur, for example, in a case in which a person has designated another by durable power of attorney to make medical decisions on his or her behalf. If the designated surrogate makes a decision that clearly threatens the patient's best interests, the decision should be overridden unless there is a clearly worded, second document executed by the patient that specifically supports the surrogate's decision. (Beauchamp and Childress 2001, 102)

Courts increasingly have been clear in stating that most decisions made by surrogates should be made in the clinical context, "at the bedside," not by the courts, and in most states a court decision is seldom necessary (Meisel 1989, 238–48; 1995, 1:237–64). Judges realize that they do not have any special competence to make this kind of decision and that usually it should be made by the family or by some other surrogate decision maker. But the law also recognizes that when a surrogate makes decisions, there are certain standards that must be followed. It has tried to ensure that the surrogate makes the decisions the patient would have made. That is, the law tries to get as close as possible to the gold standard, to the competent person's own decisions. But since the patient cannot *now* tell us what he or she wants, it is often hard, indeed, sometimes impossible, to know what those decisions would be.

STANDARDS OF SURROGATE DECISION MAKING

Since the 1985 *Conroy* case in New Jersey (*In re Conroy*), three standards—or, as Alan Meisel puts it, "a single standard with three hierarchical parts" (Meisel 1989, 279; 1995, 1:433)—have been applied to cases in which surrogates are to decide for the now-incompetent patient (Meisel 1989, 277–84; 1995, 1:432–42). *Conroy* referred to a subjective standard, a limited objective standard, and a pure objective standard. In the language often preferred by ethicists, these standards are called, respectively, "substituted judgment," "substituted judgment mixed with best interests," and "best interests."

The approach usually preferred by the courts is that the first of these (pure substituted judgment) be used if possible, followed by the second and then, only in default, the third (best interests) (Meisel 1989, 268; 1995, 1:345). Though this is understandable, I think it seldom works in the hospital setting. And I think it is often wrong.

Subjective or Substituted Judgment Standard

The subjective standard is based *only* on the subjective preferences of the patient. This presumes clear evidence of what a patient actually said she would want under specific circumstances. In a real sense, then, the more widely used term, *substituted judgment*, is misleading (Meisel 1989, 278–79; 1995, 1:433). The surrogate's own judgment is not supposed to "substitute" for that of the patient.

The surrogate is rather to decide as he or she *knows* the patient would have decided. That is what was meant by *Conroy*'s "pure subjective standard." It was supposed to be *purely subjective*, based only on the patient's known wishes. And the substituted judgment standard has come to mean this in its normal usage.

The law consistently claims a preference for this standard. This is understandable because, as we have seen, the only legal ace of trump in deciding what treatment to give and what to forgo is the contemporaneous decision of a clearly competent patient. A decision-capable competent patient tells the doctors that he or she knows that without this treatment, death will be the result. The patient chooses to forgo the treatment. Game over.

We understandably tend to think that the closest we can get to this ace of trump, when a patient is not presently able to decide, is what that person said beforehand. As I criticize the adequacy of this standard, I in no way suggest that the wishes of a competent patient should be ignored after competency is lost. For example, I have heard it suggested, in some cases in which a competent patient freely rejects a treatment that doctors or family members think should be accepted, that perhaps we might wait until the patient loses consciousness and then let the family (the surrogate decision maker) impose the treatment. This is wrong. Legally and ethically, what we have here is the decision of a competent patient, rejecting this treatment in this illness, knowing that the decision will almost certainly result in death. No one has the right to make any surrogate decision for this patient, who does not need a surrogate. But when there *is* a need for surrogate decision making, it is often hard to discern what the patient would want. And so there are difficulties connected with the substituted judgment or pure subjective standard.

The substituted judgment standard applies only to now-incompetent patients who were previously competent and expressed something about their treatment preferences. This standard cannot apply to those who were never capable of making this kind of decision, such as very young children, since they never had wishes about their treatment. But knowing the exact wishes of even a previously competent person presumes some significant amount of evidence. What is not well understood until we have experience with this kind of case is that this evidence is almost never available in the kind of precise way that is sometimes (but not always) required. Sometimes, of course, such clarity is not needed. Physicians tell the family that nothing useful or curative can be done, and the family can turn to a general treatment directive that asks that nothing be done if there is no realistic hope of a cure. In effect, the advance directive says, "Please don't do stupid stuff to me." In this kind of case, the treatment directive can be of great help in assuaging family guilt. The ethicist or the chaplain can explain to the family that they need not worry that they are doing too little to help the dying patient or failing in their responsibilities, since this is what the patient would have wanted and it is the best way to help him or her. In these cases, the general treatment directive is very helpful. But it is not the precision of the directive that is essential, it is that the directive helps the family deal with the emotional difficulty of letting go. I will discuss advance directives in the next chapter.

In some cases, we want to know the precise wishes of the patient. With any given treatment, physicians may disagree over the probability of its success and over the quality-of-life outcomes after that treatment. One doctor thinks there is a 10 percent chance of full recovery to the patient's base state, another says 30 percent, a third says the treatment can actually improve on the base state but that there is a 50 percent chance it will not work at all and a 35 percent chance that it will keep the patient alive in a reduced base state. What to do now?

Very few of us can anticipate what disease, if any, we will get, what treatments might be available to us, what prognosis and probabilities physicians will present to our surrogates, or even what we ourselves would decide in that impossible-to-anticipate situation, as empirical research is now suggesting (Fagerlin and Schneider 2004, 33–35). We may think we know what we would want if we were given the choice of a nursing home or death, but when actually faced with this kind of decision, many of us change our minds (for such a case, see Neher 2004). We may think we know that we would not like to go on living if we could not recognize our relatives, but when we see happy people in nursing homes in precisely this state, interacting with their environment in an admittedly reduced way but still interested in living, we are perhaps not so sure we want to let them die of curable pneumonia.

So the first standard, the one given legal preference, is often far less helpful than we would like it to be. Even when a patient has a written treatment directive, it will need to be interpreted, and there is no simple way to make sure it will be interpreted as the patient would have wanted were he or she able to make the decision in the present circumstances. Indeed, for this and other reasons, some bioethicists are now claiming that treatment directives are not worth the cost and should be abandoned except in situations in which clarity is possible (Fagerlin and Schneider 2004). As I have noted, I think that treatment directives can help families make these decisions, especially by alleviating guilt, and thus I do not support the claim that they should be abandoned altogether. But as I will emphasize in the next chapter, treatment directives are not exact blueprints and need interpretation.

Mixed Subjective and Objective Standard

The second standard from *Conroy*, the so-called limited objective standard, presumes that there is some evidence about what a patient would want but not, by itself, sufficient evidence on which to base a decision. Thus objective criteria concerning the best interests of the patient have to be used as well.

Pure Objective or Best Interests Standard

The so-called pure objective standard assumes that there is no evidence at all about what an incompetent patient would want; the decision is made according to the patient's best interests.

Conroy

The legal standards suggested in *Conroy* have been referred to and applied in varying ways by different courts. As we have seen, however, most have preferred to rank them in the order proposed in *Conroy*. We are supposed to look first at the purely subjective wishes of the patient, what we know from previous evidence. Only if this test fails are we to turn to the objective best interests of the patient. I have argued that in daily hospital practice this pure subjective standard is seldom available. I am therefore convinced that in almost all cases the objective best interests of the patient must be considered. This means that the first pillar, the distinction between morally ordinary and morally extraordinary treatment, does indeed come into play when surrogates make decisions for incompetent patients.

Thus *in almost all cases, surrogates may not legally or ethically choose to reject treatment that is in the objective best interests of the patient.* I may have the right, as an anti-appendectomist, to reject the appendectomy. But my family cannot reject it for me unless they have what I would want to call overwhelming evidence that I would have made that fateful choice for myself. In my judgment, it is not enough for them to know that I was a member of the Old Irish Anti-Appendectomists. They have to present clear, perhaps even overwhelming, evidence that I would have made this judgment in this case, faced now with the likelihood of dying for my beliefs. And judging by hospital experience, this kind of evidence is seldom available.

Courts have been trying to deal with this question. What weight of evidence is needed if a surrogate is to decide to reject a treatment? Is there any difference if the treatment is "objectively" beneficial to the patient? Do we need more evidence of the patient's wishes if the treatment is beneficial—it will probably make the patient better—than we do if it is not? Suppose a ventilator keeps a patient alive while doctors try to determine what has caused his or her illness, and that the illness, once discovered, is reversible and the patient can go home cured. What if the family tells the doctor that the patient told them never to use a breathing machine? Is this enough evidence to let this person die? Clearly, it is not enough evidence. But if we require too much evidence in the *other* kind of case—the more usual case in which a family agrees with doctors that further treatment is not humanly beneficial to the patient—then we face the opposite problem and we impose too much unreasonable treatment on dying patients.

Thus there are problems regarding how much evidence the law requires and as to whether or not the objective diagnosis and prognosis count. I will turn now to how the courts are dealing with these problems. I will look first, and in depth, at the *Cruzan* decision, the first case of this kind to be heard by the U.S. Supreme Court in which the proposed treatment was, by any reasonable standard, morally extraordinary. How much evidence of the patient's wishes must surrogates have before they can get the treatment stopped? Second, I will look more briefly at two cases of the other type, cases in which state courts ordered treatment continued because it was considered beneficial to the patient even though the surrogates wanted it stopped. And third, I will turn to the case of Theresa Marie "Terri" Schiavo, which has caused so much controversy. It seems that courts are coming to recognize that when surrogates make the decision, the objective best interests of the patient really do count.

CRUZAN

In 1990, when Nancy Cruzan was in her early thirties, her case was decided by the Supreme Court (*Cruzan v. Director*, 1990). For more than six years she had been in a persistent vegetative state as a result of an automobile accident. She was in a state hospital in Mount Vernon, Missouri, hooked up to a feeding tube that kept her alive. Her parents asked for permission to remove the tube. In most states, as I have noted, this could have been done at the bedside without a court order. But in Missouri, disagreement over with-drawal of the tube resulted in a court hearing.

The circuit court granted the parents' request, but the state of Missouri appealed to the Missouri Supreme Court, which in a four-to-three decision overturned the lower court and ruled that Nancy Cruzan could not be taken off the feeding treatment. Her parents, with the support of many *amicus curiae* briefs, appealed to the U.S. Supreme Court. The case was decided on June 25, 1990.

What Might Have Happened

When the *Cruzan* case was appealed to the Supreme Court, there were a number of possible directions the Court might have taken. One helpful way to illustrate the importance of this case is to spec-ulate on what the Court might have decided and to assess the im-plications of those possible rulings. *Cruzan* is now established in law, but when the case was being heard, there was considerable worry among health care providers that the decision might do great harm to the way decisions about forgoing treatment are made.

The worst outcome would have occurred had the Court con-nected this case with the abortion issue and used it as a way to establish an extreme constitutional interest in defense of life by misapplying to this issue a right-to-life interpretation of the Con-stitution. To do this, the Court might have insisted that no life-sustaining treatment could ever be forgone. Or it might have al-lowed the forgoing of treatment only for competent patients and might have refused it for all others. This move toward a more vi-talistic posture would have been possible in *Cruzan* without directly overturning *Roe v. Wade,* the 1973 abortion decision with which the *Cruzan* case has often been unfortunately linked. Courts are usually slow to overturn their prior decisions directly, and this might have offered the Court a chance to move in this direction without a direct repudiation of its earlier ruling.

As I have noted, Missouri decided as it did in *Cruzan* because of its stand as a right-to-life state. It was also Missouri that sent the Supreme Court the *Webster* case (*Webster v. Reproductive Health Services*, 1989), in which the Supreme Court did move in a more conservative direction away from some previous interpretations of *Roe v. Wade*. In addition, some among the right-to-life movement, though by no means all, have tied the two issues together, insisting that states have an absolute interest in preserving life, an interest that requires them to institute laws against all or almost all abortion and against all or almost all cessation of life-sustaining medical treatment.

That the Court did not choose this direction is probably due to a number of reasons. First, the abortion controversy concerns two beings, the pregnant woman and the fetus. All recognize the woman to be a human being, and many claim personhood for the fetus, but in *Cruzan* there is no question of a second person being harmed. Second, Nancy Cruzan, like all patients with her condition, could never be conscious; in most cases the fetus, if not aborted, would grow to live a sapient, sentient, meaningful human life. Third, and perhaps most important from the Catholic perspective, the tradition of the Roman Catholic Church is, as we have seen, best understood as permitting the forgoing of Cruzan's treatment. We will return to the specific issue of feeding tubes in chapter 6, but from what we have already seen, we can say that a treatment that yields no real human benefit is morally extraordinary. Thus official Catholic moral theology should have been in favor of overturning the Missouri Supreme Court's decision and permitting withdrawal of treatment, though some bishops and theologians, misinterpreting their tradition, disagreed. In the abortion issue, the official teaching of the Catholic Church clearly states that all direct abortions are morally wrong, though many Catholics, including a number of Catholic moral theologians, hold that this judgment cannot be absolute.

The difference between these two judgments in Catholic ethics is based on the distinction discussed in chapter 2 between killing and allowing to die. Abortion, when it is a killing, that is, when it is a direct abortion, is always wrong, according to traditional Catholic moral theology. But when abortion is an allowing to die, as in so-called indirect abortions (for example, in hysterectomies as cure for uterine cancer of pregnant women, or in some procedures as treatment of ectopic pregnancy), it is permitted. In the *Cruzan* case, since there is no question of killing, forgoing treatment is not contrary to Catholic tradition.

For all these reasons, and doubtless for its own reasons as well, the U.S. Supreme Court did not choose to rule that life-sustaining medical treatment must always be maintained in cases like Cruzan's.

A second possible outcome, one with equally disastrous potential, was that the Court might have thrown the issue back to the states for state-by-state regulation. Some states might then have ruled that nutrition and hydration must never be forgone, even by competent patients. Or they might have ruled that no life-sustaining treatment at all can be forgone, that surrogates can never choose to forgo such treatment, that though such treatment can be withheld, it can never be withdrawn, and so on. As I have already noted, most states have decided that there is no need for laws on this issue, that decisions can be made by the patient or the surrogate; state legislatures need not design detailed legislation. The Supreme Court did not open the door to the chaos that such a decision might well have brought.

The best decision, in my judgment, would have been for the Court to overturn the Missouri decision and with it the Missouri law, thus upholding the right of surrogates to refuse morally extraordinary treatment. Unfortunately, the Court rejected this direction as well. But though it did not make that decision, it did avoid the worst of its possible options.

The Decision

The *Cruzan* decision is a complicated one containing both good and bad news. This doubtless accounts for the varied reactions the decision received in the media and from ethicists, jurists, and health care professionals. Those who feared a disaster were pleased; those who hoped for the right decision were disappointed.

First, the good news. The Court upheld the right of competent people to refuse medical treatment and based this on the Fourteenth Amendment to the U.S. Constitution. The Court ruled that medical nutrition and hydration are indeed medical treatment and may rightly be forgone. It ruled that withdrawing does not differ from withholding. It pointed to the right of competent people to write living wills and implied that these directives must be followed when they provide clear and convincing evidence of a patient's wishes. And it suggested the importance of durable power of attorney (DPA) laws, such that a competent person might hand over decision-making authority to another (I will return to these advance directives in the next chapter).

In thus ruling, the Court established for the first time a nationwide legal right to forgo medical treatment. Eight of the nine justices, with the exception of Antonin Scalia, who claimed that refusing treatment is suicide (Annas 1996, 187), concurred in this, establishing the likelihood that the decision will not be overturned by a later one. This is in keeping with the emerging American consensus. It is good law and good ethics.

But there is bad news as well. In a five-to-four decision, the Court ruled that states *may* require clear and convincing evidence that patients had wished life-sustaining treatment to be forgone before surrogates may choose to forgo it. This applies not only in cases in which the treatment can be argued to be in the objective best interests of the patient, but in *all* cases. On this basis, the Supreme Court upheld the Missouri decision refusing to allow Cruzan's nutrition to be stopped, and it upheld as well the Missouri law requiring clear and convincing evidence of a patient's wishes.

This part of the decision is misguided. The dissenting opinions of Justices William Brennan and John Paul Stevens accurately demonstrate the potential for harm that this decision could bring if other states were to join Missouri in requiring clear and convincing evidence of patient wishes. In this respect the majority opinion, written by Justice William Rehnquist, is seriously flawed. And the opinion of Justice Scalia, who equated refusal of treatment with suicide, and who would have had our nation reverse the emerging consensus in radical ways, is quite simply outrageous.

But what is so problematic about allowing states to require "clear and convincing evidence"? It certainly seems reasonable. As Justice Rehnquist points out, decisions to forgo treatment are not reversible. If the requirement for clear and convincing evidence can be met by advance directives such as living wills and durable powers of attorney, why is this such a problem?

The problem is twofold. First, "clear and convincing evidence" is the highest standard of evidence that the law can require in civil matters. If states were to move toward restrictive laws requiring irrational levels of clear and convincing evidence, most of us would be unable to meet the criteria. Most people who write living wills cannot accurately foresee which diseases they will encounter and which precise sets of treatments they will want forgone in which medical circumstances. We can write general directives, but these might not meet the requirements of clear and convincing evidence.

Second, the poor and uneducated among us, and possibly the young and the old, could be disenfranchised from the right guaranteed to the rest of us. Poor people will not hire lawyers to help them through the potential maze. Medicare and Medicaid do not reimburse physicians for counseling patients on this question. On this issue, the five justices of the majority were remote from real people in real situations. Clinical experience demonstrates that most people do not have living wills and durable powers of attorney. Loving relatives make treatment decisions for them. If states were to insist on clear and convincing evidence, many Americans would be forced to endure useless and costly medical treatment. And though Justice Rehnquist is right when he says that decisions to forgo treatment are not reversible, state requirements of evidentiary hurdles are not reversible either. Patients like Nancy Cruzan would be forced irreversibly into useless death-prolonging treatments, becoming pawns of technology.

I have noted the disadvantages of having decisions like these made by the judicial system. Research by Steven Miles and Allison August lends further support to the position that these decisions are best made by patient, family, and health care team in the clinical setting. Miles and August present evidence of sexist bias in judges' decisions concerning patient choices to forgo treatment (Miles and August 1990); courts are more likely to accept such choices when men make them. In twelve of fourteen cases studied by Miles and August involving women, courts decided there was insufficient evidence of their choice, whereas only two out of eight men failed similar evidentiary requirements. Requirements of clear and convincing evidence would exacerbate this sexism, since they would necessitate constant involvement of state legislatures and courts to determine whether or not the precise requirements have been met.

The majority on the Supreme Court feared that relatives might not always act in the patient's best interests, and there is, as I have said, some justification for this fear. But it ought not be the basis for insisting that *all* surrogate decisions to forgo life-sustaining treatment require clear and convincing evidence of the patient's wishes. It is this part of the decision, and of the Missouri law, that is seriously flawed. The solution is not to require a largely unachievable level of evidence for *all* cases but to insist that the decisions reached by surrogates take account of the objective best interests of the patient. This is not as dangerous as some might claim. Doctors and other medical professionals make these kinds of decisions all the time. When they decide that a treatment will be humanly beneficial to a patient, that decision and the knowledge on which it is based has to count. If the surrogate is convinced that these particular doctors are wrong, the surrogate can always get a second or third opinion. But if there is a general agreement among physicians that treatment has a clear chance of being beneficial to the patient, this has to be considered. *Surrogates may not (ordinarily) forgo treatment when that treatment is in the objective best interests of the patient.* Thus if a treatment is to be forgone, it must be clear that the treatment is morally extraordinary, that is, it must be of little benefit or must impose a significant burden that outweighs its benefit. These restrictions, coupled with civil and criminal laws that can be brought to bear in cases in which surrogates decide to forgo treatment out of malice or greed, are already sufficient to prevent an outbreak of the criminal behavior the justices fear.

Nor is there any evidence that this kind of crime occurs with any regularity. As I will note in chapter 8, conflicts today arise more often when physicians want to stop treatment and family members want to continue it than the other way around. There is simply no reason to require the kind of evidence of the patient's own wishes that the Supreme Court has allowed states to require. To this extent, the Court's decision is a bad one.

The harm that might result from the decision, however, is only potential. Indeed, the decision to allow states to require clear and convincing evidence of a patient's wishes before surrogates can forgo treatment need have no effect at all on the consensus I have been describing. At the present time, only a few states—New York features prominently among them (Meisel 1989, 255; 1995, 1:43–44, 271–76)—have developed laws or legal precedents that seem to require this kind of evidence when the decision is made, as it should be, at the bedside. The evidentiary standard is more likely to be applied only in judicial review (Meisel 1989, 254). Though the legal variations among states and even within states are complex, hospital experience suggests that in most states and in most cases there is no need for "clear and convincing evidence" of a patient's wish before a surrogate can ask that unreasonable or morally extraordinary treatment be forgone. And there appears to be movement, even in those few states that do have such requirements, to come more in line with the general agreement not to require such hurdles (Meisel 1995, 1:43–44, 239–46).

In *Cruzan*, the Supreme Court merely upheld an existing Missouri law. It did not require such a law on the federal level or insist that other states pass similar laws. With proper understanding on the part of state legislatures, unnecessary and harmful laws requiring clear and convincing evidence of prior patient wishes to forgo burdensome or nonbeneficial treatment will not be enacted.

One final note on *Cruzan*. The case continues to be misunderstood. While the Court said that states *may* require clear and convincing evidence of a previously competent patient's wishes, it is often said that the decision *requires* this standard. For example, in an article published in 2002 in *Ethics and Medics*, the director of the Linacre Institute at the Catholic Medical Association states concerning *Cruzan* that the decision "established precedents for the states in their determination of who can refuse treatment for incompetent individuals. The court held that there should be clear and convincing evidence of the patient's wishes" (Diamond 2002, 4). This is simply false.

What happened to Nancy Cruzan? It is interesting to note that even though the Supreme Court upheld Missouri's law, the state of Missouri decided shortly thereafter not to continue to insist on feeding her. When her parents again asked the local court for permission to withdraw the feeding tube, the state announced it would have no objection. The state's attorney general's office declared that the reason for this turnabout was that further evidence had been found about Nancy Cruzan's own wishes. A few friends came forward to say that she had mentioned how she would not want this kind of useless treatment. This was enough, said the state, to meet the "clear and convincing evidence" requirement. But the same kind of testimony had been offered from the start (though not from these new sources). The real reason for the state's change of heart seems to have been that the people of Missouri were angry about the state's position and there was an election coming up. In the absence of state opposition, the judge agreed with the family. Feeding was stopped and Nancy Cruzan died on December 26, 1990 (Meisel 1995, 1:44–45).

CATHOLIC CONTROVERSY OVER Cruzan

During the course of the *Cruzan* appeal, Catholic pastoral leaders and theologians took widely divergent positions. An exploration of these positions may be helpful in furthering our understanding of the issues and serve as a review of the relationship between Catholic moral theology and U.S. law and thus as a study of the relationship among the three pillars supporting the present American consensus on forgoing treatment.

The Problem

I have argued, and will argue in greater detail in chapter 6, that Catholic tradition judges the forgoing of nutrition in cases like that of Nancy Cruzan to be morally right. Despite this fact, there has been considerable controversy in the U.S. Catholic Church over this case. The reason for this controversy is best understood by looking once again at the three pillars on which the currently emerging American consensus concerning forgoing treatment has been based. The disagreement is based on the fact, as we have often noted, that there is theoretical controversy concerning the relationship between the first two pillars, the "moral" ones, and the third, the "legal" one, that is, between the two pillars that come from Catholic moral theology (the ordinary/extraordinary distinction and the killing/allowing to die distinction) and the pillar that comes from Anglo-Saxon common law and/or from U.S. constitutional law (the concepts of liberty, privacy, and autonomy).

As we have seen, this theoretical controversy has not been resolved, despite the fact that courts have been moving toward a practical resolution of this relationship in such cases. In addition, there is debate among legal scholars over whether a legal right to privacy exists in the Constitution and over how far it, or similar legal rights and freedoms, ought to extend. These debates are basic to the Catholic controversy over *Cruzan*.

Two Catholic Briefs in Cruzan

Among the *amicus curiae*, or "friend of the court," briefs submitted to the Supreme Court in the *Cruzan* case were two by official Catholic organizations.

One position is presented in the brief submitted by the United States Catholic Conference (USCC) (United States Catholic Conference 1989), the educational and research wing of the National Conference of Catholic Bishops, which argues against the request to withdraw the feeding tube.

In the brief, the bishops can not and do not appeal to their own tradition to argue that it is *morally* wrong for Cruzan's treatment to be stopped. They can not and do not claim that their own tradition rejects the right to refuse morally extraordinary treatment, treatment that is of little benefit or that, while of benefit, is of considerable burden. Nor do they claim that the continued treatment of Nancy Cruzan offers her sufficient benefit to make it an ordinary means and therefore obligatory. They do not claim that there is no burden involved, certainly to the family and to society, and, in terms of useless affliction, and thus of degradation though not of actual suffering, to Nancy Cruzan herself. Nor do they claim that their own tradition holds that the forgoing of morally extraordinary treatment is euthanasia, that is, killing. Rather, the Catholic tradition says it is allowing to die and thus is morally right in cases like Cruzan's. The bishops do not claim that they would want the law to make it illegal for surrogates to choose to forgo *other* morally extraordinary means, such as ventilation, yet they make no coherent attempt to distinguish medical nutrition from medical ventilation. They seem to be aware that their own tradition would not allow them to say that the withdrawal of Cruzan's feeding tube is immoral, though they never explicitly state what they think the morality of withdrawal in this case would be.

Nonetheless, the bishops argue that withdrawal of treatment ought to be illegal. They do so mostly because they oppose the understanding of the right to privacy and autonomy on which the legal submission by Cruzan's family was based. This, in turn, is at least partly because the bishops fear that the support of such a right to privacy will sustain the so-called right to abortion, which the church officially opposes. This is clear in the brief itself, where reference is made to abortion on demand as a result of such a right to privacy.

The bishops fear, properly I think, that an absolute stress on the right to privacy and autonomy to the detriment of the state's interest in support of life would create an imbalance not intended in the Constitution, which would support an unrestricted right to abortion and would also open the door to euthanasia. They fear that the right to privacy might support a legal right to assistance in suicide. Therefore, they opposed the Cruzans' petition to remove the feeding tube.

But this means they argue that it ought to be illegal to do what their own tradition says it is morally right to do. This is incoherent. It is also dangerous. If the decision in *Cruzan* had rejected patients' and surrogates' rights to refuse useless treatment, a likely result would have been a backlash, on both the basis of economic impossibility and the basis of human cruelty to patient and family. That backlash might very well have led to what the bishops fear, legislative action to permit euthanasia. Indeed, there is already some evidence that the *Cruzan* decision has furthered the euthanasia movement.

But a second Roman Catholic brief was submitted in the *Cruzan* case, this one by SSM Health Care System, a St. Louis–based corporation of the Franciscan Sisters of Mary, representing 130 Catholic health care facilities nationwide (SSM 1989). This brief makes all the proper distinctions and comes up with the right answer, true to Catholic tradition.

Like that of the USCC, the SSM brief argues against making absolute the right to privacy such that euthanasia might become a legal right. For the SSM, as for the USCC, sanctity of life is essential. The Constitution does not propose an absolute right to privacy or autonomy. Citizens pay taxes, for example, and we have no absolute right to keep all our earnings and do with them what we want. The common good requires sharing, even a sharing legally enacted by government. Humanly, as well as legally, there is no perfect privacy or perfect autonomy. Privacy and autonomy are unhelpful terms if they are taken to imply a reductionist isolated individualism. Informed consent, a medical ethical process based on the notion of patient autonomy, does not presuppose that the patient makes decisions free from all sources of social influence. This notion of privacy and autonomy is neither possible nor desirable. In arguing against absolutist interpretations of the right to privacy and autonomy, the USCC and the SSM briefs are in agreement.

But unlike the USCC brief, the SSM brief properly points out that in the *Cruzan* case the withdrawal of treatment is the withdrawal of extraordinary means and is not euthanasia. It insists that beneficial (or morally ordinary) treatment may not legally or morally be withheld by surrogate decision makers, a position with which the courts have generally agreed. It insists on the importance of the benefit-burden analysis. It argues against the two extremes mentioned in chapter 1, the extreme of insisting that everything be done to preserve biological life and the extreme of disregarding the importance of physical life altogether. It is, in sum, well written, properly reflective of the Catholic tradition, and the basis for good law.

There remains the question of what to do about those who are capable of making decisions yet reject morally ordinary treatment. Should their decision be made illegal? Should they be forced to have treatment? I think the present agreement of the courts that those capable of making these decisions be allowed to refuse any and all medical treatment (that adult Jehovah's Witnesses, for example, be allowed to refuse blood transfusions) is morally correct. But I recognize that this is an area where Catholic tradition and U.S. law may be seen, in some interpretations, to disagree. In the *Cruzan* case, however, there is no such point of contention. Catholic tradition is clear that Cruzan's treatment may rightly be forgone, since it is the forgoing of morally extraordinary means, which is ethically right, and since it is allowing to die and not euthanasia.

Conclusions on *Cruzan*

The *Cruzan* case concerns the petition of a surrogate to withdraw morally extraordinary treatment. In this kind of case, the laws of most states permit that decision to be made at the bedside by surrogates in communication with the medical team. But what are the courts doing about cases in which surrogates decide to withhold or withdraw treatment that the medical team or someone else claims to be truly beneficial? What role does the best interests standard play? Fortunately, the position that I and others have been advocating is gaining legal support. I turn now to a brief look at two cases of this kind.

Martin and *Wendland* and the Emerging Consensus

State laws differ on the quality of evidence needed before surrogates are allowed to forgo treatment for a patient. But there is growing judicial agreement about what to do when it seems that the treatment may be of benefit to the patient and surrogates claim that they know the patient would not have wanted it. Cases like these are difficult because the degree of benefit from the treatment and the kind of life the patient is leading vary from case to case and are interpreted differently by different people. Still, it seems that courts are beginning to recognize that the substituted judgment standard does not trump the best interests standard after all. Even in states where clear and convincing evidence of a patient's wishes is, quite rightly, not required when surrogates decide to forgo morally extraordinary treatment, courts are not allowing them to forgo beneficial treatment unless it is clear that the patient said that he or she did not want it.

Martin v. Martin

In the *Martin* case, heard in Michigan in 1995, the patient's brain was damaged in a car accident. The Michigan court refused to allow his wife to withdraw the feeding tube even though she claimed he had told her he would not want to be kept on machines. The court almost certainly did this because Martin was still able to interact with his surroundings to some extent. Interpreted one way, it might seem that Michigan, by this ruling, has joined New York and Missouri as states requiring clear and convincing evidence when surrogates want to forgo treatment (Meisel 2003, 13–15). If so, this would be unfortunate. But as Alan Meisel points out, "It is essential to note that the court intimated that the holding . . . might not apply to patients more seriously injured than Martin, specifically, patients in a P.V.S. [persistent vegetative state]" (Meisel 2003, 15). I do not wish to defend the court's specific conclusion in this case—I do not know enough about Martin's condition—and I certainly would not want the forgoing of treatment without clear and convincing evidence to be limited to PVS patients. But I do think the general direction of the decision is right in that it supports the legal importance of the objective best interests standard. Substituted judgment does not automatically supersede best interests.

Wendland v. Wendland

In California in 2001, Robert Wendland was severely brain damaged in a car accident. He was incontinent, paralyzed, and on a feeding tube. But he was able to interact and to respond to simple commands. Three family members told the court he had told them that he would not want to be kept alive in this kind of circumstance. They claimed that he had said this often and strongly. When they asked the hospital to remove the feeding tube, an ethics consultation was called and the ethics committee agreed to the withdrawal. But two other family members opposed this and obtained a restraining order. Two California courts decided in effect that the patient's best interests required that nutrition not be withdrawn. The California Supreme Court determined that a standard of evidence less rigorous than "clear and convincing evidence" of a patient's wishes is enough to allow the forgoing of treatment when the patient is terminally ill or permanently unconscious, but that in cases like *Wendland* there has to be clear and convincing evidence that this patient would not want this treatment in this circumstance. The best interest standard counts.

Again, here I do not claim to concur with the actual decision—I simply do not know enough about Robert Wendland's condition.[1] But I have served on ethics consultations when this kind of issue was at stake. Such cases, in which patients have suffered from strokes or other brain injuries leading to severe mental impairment, are commonplace. I recall two cases that were somewhat like *Martin* and *Wendland*. In one of these, the consultation team decided that the patient's condition—there was no interaction with the environment at all, though she was not technically in PVS—warranted the family's request to forgo continued nutrition and hydration. In the other case, where the patient was still able to interact in a happy if significantly restricted way, the team decided that the feeding should not be forgone. Some have told me that the correct decision should have been to maintain feeding for both, that the team did not sufficiently value life. Others have suggested that nutrition should have been withdrawn from both, that the team was too vitalistic and did not pay sufficient attention to what the families wanted or to what they said they knew about the patients' wishes. And, of course, still others agree with what was done. This kind of judgment is not always easy. But it is clear that neither the substituted judgment standard nor the best interests standard can be seen in isolation. In almost all cases, both the prior wishes of the patient (substituted judgment/subjective standard) and the patient's present condition and the possible outcome of treatments (best interests/objective standard) have to be considered. Substituted judgment does not deserve the automatic hierarchy over best interests that some court decisions have given it.

But this does not mean that the wishes of previously competent people are insignificant. One of the ways patients can help ensure that these wishes will be carried out is by advance directives. I will discuss these in the next chapter.

The Schiavo *Case*

The case of Theresa Marie "Terri" Schiavo offers a further look at whether or not a surrogate's wishes to forgo treatment ought to be honored. The case became well known, even notorious, and carried political, legal, and ethical implications. In this section I will introduce the case and briefly suggest its legal implications for honoring surrogate decisions. In chapter 6, I will return to it in the context of recent debates in Catholic bioethics.

On February 25, 1990, Theresa Marie Schiavo suffered cardiac arrest, which resulted in a loss of oxygen to her brain. All tests taken then and thereafter showed that she was in a persistent (permanent) vegetative state (Quill 2005, 1630). I will return to a fuller description of this condition in chapter 6, and for the moment note only that PVS means a total lack of capacity for inner or outer awareness. PVS patients cannot dream, pray, suffer, or experience thoughts, emotions, or feelings of any kind. They do exhibit movement and their eyes do open and close and wander about, which is often misunderstood, especially by family members, as attempts to communicate (Schiavo was frequently shown on television this way). But these movements are completely involuntary and not in response to the environment.

After eight years of caring for his wife in this condition, Michael Schiavo decided to ask that the feeding tube be removed. Members of his wife's family objected. Two Florida courts found clear and convincing evidence that she was in PVS and that she would not want continued treatment were she able to decide (note the importance here of the objective, best interests standard; there was no advance directive and evidence of her wishes was not entirely clear). The Florida Supreme Court declined to review that decision (Annas 2005, 1711).

But because of objections from family members who claimed they had new evidence of her condition and new treatment options, another court hearing took place in 2003 (*In re Guardianship of Schiavo*). Again the court agreed with Schiavo's husband and again the Florida Supreme Court refused to hear an appeal (Annas 2005, 1711–12). Family members, with support from some religious and political groups, then asked the Florida legislature to enact a law requiring that the feeding be continued, which they did in passing "Terri's Law" in October 2003. The law was drawn up in such a way that it applied only to Schiavo and to no one else (Annas 2005, 1712). In the fall of 2004 the Florida Supreme Court ruled this law to be unconstitutional because it was an encroachment by the legislative branch onto the judicial branch of government (*Bush v. Schiavo*). The U.S. Supreme Court refused to hear the case, and the feeding tube was removed on March 18, 2005.

In a final attempt to maintain the feeding tube, Congress reconvened from Easter recess for the precise purpose of enacting a law concerning Theresa Schiavo. Annas correctly notes the "uninformed and frenzied rhetoric" that was part of the debate in Congress (Annas 2005, 1713). A number of Republican physician-members of Congress claimed to be sure that she was not in PVS, a claim that would be refuted when an autopsy after her death showed clear evidence that that indeed had been her condition. The law Congress passed, which was signed by President George W. Bush on March 21, in effect it required a federal court to hear the case. The following day the federal court ruled. Judge James D. Whittemore, U.S. District Court, refused to order the feeding tube to be reinserted (*Schiavo ex rel. Schindler v. Schiavo*) (Annas 2005, 1713–14). Theresa Marie Schiavo died, still unconscious, on March 31, 2005, more than fifteen years after her last conscious experience.

In the aftermath of this case, with all its attendant publicity, one conclusion commonly drawn was the need to make one's wishes clear in written advance directives (Dombi 2005). Had Terri Schiavo done this, it was said, the strife and the drawn-out court battles would not have occurred. But when I return to discuss treatment directives in the next chapter, we will discover significant reasons why they often do not in fact provide the resolution that is sought. In my judgment, the principle legal conclusion to be drawn from this unfortunate case is, as Rebecca Dresser claims (Dresser 2005), that there is a need for some sort of objective standard in the law. Dresser points to *Martin, Wendland,* and *Schiavo* as three cases proving this need (Dresser 2005, 21). And this is precisely what I have been arguing for in this chapter. The pure subjective standard (the pure substituted judgment standard), to which courts have all too often given preference, is insufficient. Regarding the *Schiavo* case, Dresser writes:

> Much of the opposition to the Florida court rulings was based on weaknesses in the substituted judgment standard. The testimony about Ms. Schiavo's previous statements was general enough to raise doubts about whether she would indeed have refused nutrition and hydration. And years after her brain injury, with her family so divided, could anyone really know what she would decide if she were, in the language of the *Quinlan* court, "miraculously lucid for an interval . . . and perceptive of her irreversible condition"? (Dresser 2005, 20)

In *Schiavo,* it is clear that objective evidence *was* considered by the courts and that they properly judged the decision of her husband Michael to remove the feeding tube to be the right one.

Deciding for the Never Competent

The issues we have discussed apply to patients who once were able to make decisions and now no longer can. In these cases, surrogates need to look at both the patients' previously expressed wishes and their best interests. In cases of young children or others who, perhaps because of a lifelong mental deficiency, have never been able to make or express autonomous wishes about treatment, the situation is in many ways easier. In such cases it is clear that only the best interests standard (pure objective standard) ought to apply. It is sometimes argued that parents and other family members may rightly include their own interests in this decision, but this is not generally accepted and has never been sanctioned by courts. Although it is perfectly normal for family members to consider their interests to some extent, health care providers would never be justified in acting contrary to the clear best interests of a child or a never-competent person.

The paradigmatic case here is that of the young child whose Jehovah's Witness parents ask that a lifesaving blood transfusion not be given. In such cases, courts have consistently overruled the parents, and in emergency situations it is clear that physicians must transfuse (Meisel 1989, 417–21; 1995, 2:283–89). In emergency cases, it may be possible to get a court order over the telephone, but even if this is not done, emergency transfusion is required. The clear best interests of the child prevail legally and ethically. When the benefit and the necessity of the treatment are less clear, however, courts are not as quick to override parental refusal (Meisel 1989, 417–21; 1995, 2:283–89).

Yet we need to be especially aware that the best interests of a child or of an incompetent patient are not limited to the physical or medical. The child will return to his or her family and will have to live with them. If they now reject the child, even unconsciously, because he or she has in their minds been tainted, this is contrary to the child's best interests. If an alternative treatment is likely to be successful, it should be considered.

A Hip for a Jehovah's Witness

I was asked to consult on a case in which a child of Jehovah's Witness parents needed a new hip. He was chronologically an adult but suffered from moderately severe retardation. The orthopedic surgeon told us that it was likely he would need to be transfused as part of the surgery and said he would not perform the surgery unless permission were given for transfusion. We quickly reached the "right" conclusion that the best interests of the patient meant we needed to override the parents' objection. But a sensitive and very "streetwise" social worker was not so quick to agree. He pointed out to us that the patient might indeed be harmed by the transfusion—not medically, but socially and psychologically. After all, family cohesion is important. So he called neighboring hospitals and found a surgeon who told us he knew that in this case he could do the work without the need for blood. He informed the parents of this, and they gladly went elsewhere for the surgery. Sometimes book answers are not the right ones. It is also sometimes the case that Jehovah's Witnesses will refuse the transfusion of whole blood but will accept certain blood products or even autologous transfusion of stored blood. Imagination and sensitivity are valuable attributes for those who serve on ethics committees.

NOTE

1. If the facts in the case are properly interpreted by Lawrence Nelson, the attorney who represented Robert Wendland's wife, Rose, who wanted the treatment stopped, then it does seem that continued feeding may not have been in Robert's best interests (Nelson 2003). Though Wendland was not technically in PVS, Nelson claims that he was very close to that condition, as his interaction was minimal at best. And though the court found he was not terminally ill, he did indeed die (of pneumonia), despite ongoing treatment, three weeks before the court issued its decision. Nelson rightly argues that the court's requirement of clear and convincing evidence, despite the exception the court made for PVS and for terminal illness (Dresser 2002, 10), may well be too stringent. Surrogates ought to be able to forgo treatment that is not in the patient's best interests even when there is no clear and convincing evidence of what the patient would have wanted, and this ought not be limited to permanent unconsciousness

or terminal illness in the legal sense. I have made this very argument in this chapter in the context of the *Cruzan* case. So the actual decision in the *Wendland* case may have been wrong. Courts are not the best venue for this kind of complex decision. But I support the fact that courts are beginning to recognize that the best interests standard does count even when surrogates claim they know what the patient would have wanted, though in this case the court may well have misunderstood what that standard means.

In line with this, some legal scholars are beginning to criticize the all-too-often automatic preference given to autonomy over beneficence. Carl E. Schneider (2004) issues what he calls a "cri de coeur" (heartfelt cry) about this in a brief piece on a court decision to allow autonomy to override the best interests of a schizophrenic patient who refused medication. He laments that "from the start . . . 'individual rights' and 'autonomy' exude the odor of sanctity, while 'state interests' and 'beneficence' trail the stench of paternalism, even tyranny" (10). Bioethics is best served when it serves its patients, which requires considering beneficence (the best interests standard) along with autonomy (the substituted judgment standard) rather than giving automatic precedence to autonomy.

Chapter 5

Advance Directives

AN *advance directive* is an instruction made in advance by a competent person specifying what that person wants if and when he or she should become ill and unable to make treatment decisions. There are two kinds of advance directives: proxy directives and treatment directives. *Proxy directives* appoint someone to make decisions if a person no longer can do so. *Treatment directives* (often called "living wills") are instructions, usually in writing, about what kind of care a person would want. Because I think proxy directives are often more helpful than treatment directives, I will begin with them.

PROXY DIRECTIVES

A proxy directive, sometimes called a durable power of attorney for health care, is a document by which a person appoints a surrogate decision maker. States have different laws concerning these. Some may require that they be written according to some approved formula, or, as in Pennsylvania, the law may suggest a form but not impose it. A DPA refers to a legal device by which one person transfers certain authority to another. Some powers of attorney are not "durable." That is, they cease once the person authorizing them loses the capacity to decide and thus to revoke them. Powers of attorney are often granted authorizing others to take care of financial matters, deal with investments, and so on. In some cases of this sort, the person wants to be able to oversee the decisions of the one authorized to act on his or her behalf and so makes it clear that when he or she cannot do so, the power stops. In the case of health care, however, the idea is to appoint someone to make decisions when the person no longer can, so when these are called "powers of attorney," they are, in fact, "durable." They are still in effect after the person loses the capacity to revoke them. Indeed, they do not go into effect or become operative until the person loses decision-making capacity, since otherwise, as we saw in chapter 3, the person makes decisions for himself or herself. The name used, whether "health care proxy" or "durable power of attorney for health care," does not really matter; it depends on how the law of an individual state is crafted. As far as I know, all states now have some kind of law authorizing advance directives of this kind.

This approach is simpler than treatment directives and, in my judgment, has a number of advantages. One ethicist has called the proxy directive the "Committee of the Person" (Maguire 1974, 169–71). One appoints another person or, possibly but not usually, a group of people to make decisions concerning treatment in case one is unable to make such decisions for oneself. The advantages of this approach are its flexibility and its emphasis on human friendship and love. One person expresses trust in another to do what is best. No one can ever predict completely the circumstances of a particular process of dying, so this approach simply says to a family member or friend, "I trust you. Do what you think is right, what you feel I would want. I trust your motives. If you make a mistake, so be it. It is better for me to put this trust in you than in my physicians, or the courts, or even, possibly, my family."

Admittedly, the proxy directive approach is not perfect. It has its disadvantages. What of possible conflict of interest? The person I appoint might turn out later on to hate me or want my money. What of the burden this might impose on the surrogate? In this approach, as indeed in aspects of this whole question, what one thinks one will want when one is healthy and watching people dying on television can be quite different from what one actually feels and wants when dying oneself. Despite these difficulties, there is much that is humanly attractive in this approach, and to my knowledge Catholic ethicists do not oppose it. Assuming that the actions taken by the surrogate do not include active euthanasia or physician-assisted suicide, which are illegal in all states but Oregon, there is no reason for the tradition of Catholic moral theology to reject proxy directives.

The Supreme Court's *Cruzan* decision may have increased the importance of proxy directives. In her concurring opinion, Justice Sandra Day O'Connor suggested the possibility of a future Court ruling that surrogates appointed by power of attorney have exactly the same right to decide as the patient would have if capable. If the Supreme Court were to issue such a ruling, this would go beyond the consensus by allowing legally appointed surrogates to withhold humanly beneficial treatment based on substituted judgment and not requiring that such decisions be in the best interests of the patient. To date this has not happened. As we have seen, state court decisions have thus far insisted that best interests be considered. Still, the *Cruzan* decision does underline the authority of the surrogate and the importance of choosing wisely. It is clear that the Court intended to suggest the durable power of attorney as one way states might acknowledge that patients have given clear and convincing evidence of their wishes. So in the wake of *Cruzan*, and of *Schiavo*, especially in those states with strict evidence requirements such as New York and Missouri, durable powers of attorney may be patients' best bet.

Treatment Directives

The second kind of advance directive is an instruction or treatment directive, made through a document often called a living will. This is a document drawn up or a form filled out by a competent person giving instructions concerning the kind of treatment he or she wishes if and when he or she is seriously ill or injured and not able to make treatment decisions. Most treatment directives ask for a limitation of treatment, though that is not required; directives can also request aggressive treatment. There is a standard form of the type of living will that limits treatment, though there are a number of variations of it. This is the operative paragraph in the form suggested by Concern for Dying, an organization formed to help people prepare for death:

> If at such a time the situation should arise in which there is no expectation of my recovery from extreme physical or mental disability, I direct that I be allowed to die and not be kept alive by medications, artificial means, or "heroic measures." I do, however, ask that medication be mercifully administered to me to alleviate suffering even though this may shorten my remaining life.

It is clear that in this document there is no question of active euthanasia. Though the document is vague, it enables patients to express their general desires concerning treatment. It gives physicians at least a general sense of patients' wishes and says, in effect, "Don't do stupid stuff to me." The living will is morally acceptable for those who find comfort in signing one and is in keeping with the Catholic tradition.

Three points about treatment directives are very important and are sometimes overlooked. First, the absence of such a directive is not an indication that a patient wants heroic measures or morally extraordinary means of treatment. Indeed, most people do not have treatment directives. Physicians ought to discuss these matters with patients and get a sense of their wishes. This type of discussion can be begun in a nonthreatening way while the person is still healthy. Indeed, patients may initiate these discussions themselves. Because family members often discuss issues of this kind among themselves, physicians and nurses should ask them if their sick relative has talked about this. The lack of documents ought never be construed as an indication that a patient would have insisted on aggressive treatment.

Second, living wills do not always mean that patients want treatment forgone. I have presented them that way here because this is usually the reason they are used and this is the context envisioned by those who support them and by those who have crafted state legislation about them. Historically, they were developed to return the authority to forgo treatment to patients and away from doctors, who tended to insist on it. But people who make living wills are not required to say in them that they want to forgo extraordinary means or aggressive treatment. In fact, they can indicate that they *do* want such treatment. In Pennsylvania, for example, the law requires that in any statutorily enforceable treatment directive people must specify whether they do or do not want tube feeding if they are permanently unconscious. It cannot be presumed that they say no. Advance directives have to be read. It is not enough just to chart them.

Third, the fact that a person has signed a treatment directive does not mean that that person is refusing CPR in the event of cardiac arrest. It is not clear why, but it seems that when a patient indicates on admittance to a hospital that he or she has a living will, there is a tendency to assign an automatic DNR—do not resuscitate. And this happens even for patients admitted in good health for minor and curable illnesses. Somehow the terms "advance directive" and "living will" are translated in the busy hospital setting to DNR. I know one medical ethicist who denies having a living will when admitted for minor illnesses because she is afraid of just this danger.

State Laws

The issue becomes more complex when the question of statutory change in state laws is introduced. These *natural death acts* or *advance directive for health care acts* generally make legally binding (or at least legally recognize) documents similar to, but often more specific than, the living will. I think there are reasons to worry about some of this legislation, though it is now so widespread that perhaps the risks of these laws are not as serious as some ethicists initially feared.

First, natural death acts may suggest the legalization of active euthanasia (a bill introduced into the Idaho legislature, but not passed, fell into this category, and a number of initiatives have been introduced to make active euthanasia or assisted suicide legal; in Oregon, as we shall see, such an initiative is now law). Moralists who oppose active euthanasia oppose those statutes that allow this or are potentially open to that possibility.

Second, paradoxically, some natural death acts are so specific that they imply that only in this particular case or under these special circumstances can treatment be withheld or withdrawn. These bills tend to reduce, at least implicitly, the flexibility given to the families of dying, incompetent patients. In some states, for example, laws specifically ruled out the inclusion of nutrition and hydration as treatments that a person may request be forgone (this may now be illegal in light of *Cruzan*). In Pennsylvania, people who make advance directives must say whether they want tube feeding if they are terminally ill or permanently unconscious; if they fail to fill in this part of the document, they must be given this treatment if it is medically indicated. People who do not make an advance directive may be able to escape tube feeding if their family agrees. When one of my graduate students showed her living will to the class we noticed that she had filled out one section saying she did not want tube feeding but failed to check the proper box; her living will might well have been interpreted legally as meaning she had to have tube feeding, though hopefully wise doctors would understand otherwise. Nevertheless, with this kind of legislation, living wills may paradoxically increase the likelihood that treatment will be continued, either because the law forbids including the permission to forgo a certain treatment or because the document the person signs does not explicitly include a specific treatment or a particular circumstance in the general permission granted to withhold or withdraw treatment.

Third, there is the danger that those who have not signed such a document will find, precisely for that reason, that they are subjected to invasive and useless medical measures to prolong life. Physicians, and possibly courts, may assume that because a given patient never signed such a document, that patient did not want treatment withheld under any circumstances. The passing of a statute to enact a right that people already have can reduce that right by implying that the state grants it, whereas in fact it is a "natural" right, recognized as such by common law and, as I have noted, by the courts in many states. This problem is increased in those bills that require that the document be periodically renewed. What if the person fails to renew it? Does this imply that this individual wishes heroic treatment even when such treatment would ordinarily be easily forgone with the family's agreement? Does this imply that there is no evidence of the patient's wishes on which to base substituted judgment?

One way in which some state laws try to alleviate these problems is by saying explicitly, as does the Advance Directive for Health Care Act in Pennsylvania, that the law is *cumulative legislation*. That is, this new law is only an addition to the rights people already had to tell their doctors and families what treatment they would want. If people wish to take advantage of the new law, they write their directive according to its legal requirements. This "statutory" advance directive then has the advantages the law gives it, usually some degree of legal force and some degree of immunity from lawsuit to the physicians and hospitals that follow it. And it has disadvantages as well: it may only become effective under certain circumstances (in Pennsylvania, only when a person is terminally ill or in a state of permanent unconsciousness, for example) or it may need to be notarized and witnessed by a certain number of people. But if the state law is clear that the legislation is cumulative, people can still make their wishes known in other ways as well, for example, by telling their families or by writing their wishes down in another document. One of the finest treatment directives I ever saw was written on a single yellow sheet of paper by a woman who signed and dated it and gave it to her children. This was not an "operative" advance directive under Pennsylvania law, but courts, including Pennsylvania courts (*In re Fiori*, 1996), do not usually insist on statutory written documents as the only valid sources for knowledge of a patient's wishes. Even when it is clear that the legislation is cumulative, there is a natural tendency to think that because the state law has placed certain limitations on its statutory advance directives, it wants these same limitations placed on other, nonstatutory directives as well. My case experience has taught me that this is true. Medical personnel become aware of the restrictions in the law—they have to know these—and then are less sure what to do with other, nonstatutory directives that they may be ethically and legally required to consider.

Fourth, a final caution applies to any statute that, as its purpose, enables the legal allowing of death. Laws must ensure that such policies are not carried out in order to rid society of individuals it considers burdensome, financially or otherwise. The wealthy have better access to medical care facilities and scarce resources, and thus the poor and powerless are subject to earlier deaths. There is always a temptation to eliminate the poor as a way of eliminating poverty. Whatever laws are enacted, controls are essential to make sure this does not happen.

These risks, inherent in state legislation, may not be reason enough to conclude that such legislation is on the whole harmful. Whether statutorily authorized or not, treatment directives make it easier for health care professionals to know that the patient has considered these issues and made some decisions. They relieve the minds and consciences of family members, who worry what to do, and they help resolve disputes between family members who disagree about the patient's wishes. For all these reasons, living wills are probably a good idea, even if specific legislation aimed at them may be problematic.

The proxy directive allows greater flexibility than is possible with a living will. Now a trusted friend, rather than a physician or the court, will make decisions regarding medical treatment. And this approach offers something I consider theologically essential: an enhancement of human trust and of trust in God. When the "committee of the person" is made legal by a statutorily enforceable proxy directive or durable power of attorney, the person has ensured as much as is possible that flexible and humanly meaningful decisions about treatment will be carried out. Signing a general living will document is also helpful, as it supplies yet another indication of what the person wants.

Most people have not signed advance directives, but someone still needs to make decisions for them if they cannot do so themselves. Usually these decisions are made by family members, who act as surrogate decision makers for the patient. In most states (but these differ, so it is necessary to check in one's own state), when there is no proxy directive and when family members are in agreement about what should be done, there is no need for court involvement. When there is disagreement, it usually helps to wait for a time so that the family can come to agreement. Sometimes, though this is rare (cases like *Schiavio*, despite their notoriety, are exceptions to the general process), the only answer is recourse to the court.

Interpreting Treatment Directives

The law tries to get us back to the ace of trump, or as close to it as possible, when a person cannot make treatment decisions. Courts would like to have decisions of this sort be clear and precise. They usually do not want to make these judgments; they want the patient or the surrogate to make them. As we saw in the last chapter, when the patient is not able to make decisions, it is rarely possible to achieve this gold standard because people generally cannot anticipate their precise future situation. Thus the treatment directives they leave for their surrogates to follow always need "objective" interpretation. Generally, they are not enough in themselves to allow a clear decision about treatment to be made. Interpretation of the directive is helped by prior communication. Though such communication is often difficult, the earlier it occurs, the better. But communication by the person for whom decisions are going to be made should take place—first with the surrogate who is likely to help with the interpretation, whether that surrogate is chosen by DPA or proxy directive or simply by family relationship, and then with the primary care physician.

The *Conroy, Cruzan, Martin, Wendland,* and *Schiavo* cases all concerned the need to interpret a patient's wishes, and interpretation applies whether or not a patient has signed a treatment directive. In the real world of the hospital, this task is usually done by physicians and surrogates. They should take into consideration both what they know of the patient's general wishes and what they know of the medical prognosis and diagnosis. Interpretation thus always involves the objective best interests standard, whether pure or limited. There are very few cases in which a general treatment directive (the kind we make when we are basically healthy) could be sufficiently precise to authorize a surrogate to withhold or withdraw a treatment when that treatment is in the objective best interests of the patient (a directive specifying refusal for a religious reason might be an exception). So the presence of a living will does not change my claim throughout these last two chapters that the gold standard of legal decision making applies *almost only* to currently competent alert patients and *almost never* to patients who have lost the capacity to decide even if they wrote down their wishes in a treatment directive.

Exceptions to the Need for Interpretation

There are three areas of exceptions to the need for interpretation, instances in which treatment directives may give precise orders that can be followed. First, since the area of permanent unconsciousness has been analyzed and dealt with in numerous court cases, people should be urged, when writing treatment directives, to say whether or not they want to be kept alive should such a diagnosis be made. They should include whether or not they want ventilation, dialysis, antibiotics, CPR, and, most important, tube feeding.

Second, there are cases in which there is a well-established religious tradition for refusing treatment. The obvious case is that of a Jehovah's Witness who refuses blood. (Below I discuss an example in which I express my hesitation to withhold transfusion when the Jehovah's Witness is unable to make a contemporaneous decision. But a clear, well-drafted refusal in a living will might be sufficient evidence of the patient's intentions.)

Third, once a person is diagnosed with a certain disease, it then becomes easier for that person to clarify with the physician what exactly is likely to happen and what the options are—and to write down choices about those options. What do we want to call this document? We might call it a treatment directive (it is one) and even a living will, but it is not an *advance* directive at all. It is, rather, the contemporaneous decision of a competent patient faced with treatment choices about this illness with these characteristics. A patient is told that such and such will likely happen as a cancer progresses (there is seldom absolute certainty in medicine, but in many cases we can be virtually sure of a disease's progress). At some point, decision-making capacity will be lost. We already know that the cancer has metastasized; we have tried chemotherapy, and the last attempt failed. The patient is asked, "Do you want another attempt?" and replies no. "When you lose your ability to breathe unassisted, do you want a ventilator (knowing that once you are on it, you will not be able to get off)?" Again the patient replies no. In a sense, that is an advance directive, but in another sense it is the contemporaneous decision of a competent patient. *This* living will is precise enough to follow exactly.

CHECK-BOX LIVING WILLS

What about living will forms that try to anticipate different scenarios? In response to the criticism that treatment directives are too vague to be very helpful, perhaps it is possible to design treatment directives that include a number of illness scenarios and treatment options. Some are better than others. But all of them take an enormous amount of intelligent perusal and explanation before the subtle distinctions among the scenarios and treatment options are understood. In my experience, many people fill out treatment directives like these in contradictory ways. If even doctors sometimes order contradictory treatments or tests, surely we must expect laypeople to do so. At the very least, a person who considers using one of these directives should schedule a long appointment with his or her physician to go over the options in detail. Physicians are unlikely to spend hours with each of their patients talking about multiple possible future scenarios, but in the absence of such conversation, a check-box living will in all probability will fail at describing the person's wishes and, if followed, may even be dangerous (Fagerlin and Schneider 2004, 34–35).

Thus treatment directives almost always need interpretation. The better a health care institution is at this, the more it has well-trained ethicists aboard, the more it has a good pastoral care department, and the better it is at understanding cultural diversity among patients and surrogate decision makers, the better that hospital or nursing home will be at understanding and carrying out patients' wishes.

Two Examples

Two fictionalized cases in which it might seem that a patient's wishes have been precisely expressed but in which, perhaps, there is still room for hesitation will serve to illustrate this. I am placing both cases in Pennsylvania, allowing me to fill in some actual legal details to make the cases more accurate.

Curable Pneumonia

The first case is based on an event said to have occurred in eastern Pennsylvania. A man wrote in his treatment directive that he did not, under any circumstances, want to be intubated or put on a mechanical ventilator. He checked the no box in every single section that mentioned a ventilator. He signed it, had it notarized, and carried it in his briefcase. He told his wife, his children, his doctor, and his malpractice lawyer that he never wanted a ventilator. Then he got pneumococcal pneumonia. The paramedics who came to his house with the ambulance found him gasping for breath and took him to the ER. His wife and his children went with him. The physicians said they could cure him almost certainly with antibiotics and that he would be home and well in a week or ten days. But as the bacteria were now suppressing his respiration, they needed to put him on a ventilator for a few days while the antibiotics worked their medical miracle. But his wife and children pointed to the treatment directive. The physicians agreed not to intubate. And the man died.

Most who have heard of this case agree that he died because no one had the sense to realize that what he meant was "no ventilator when it means that I will lie in bed terminally ill for months on that machine as my mother did." This man died because procedural justice took precedence over substantive good.

In most states where there are laws about treatment directives, the law says that a treatment directive does not become operative until the person is *both* unable to make decisions *and* terminally ill. In Pennsylvania, one must be either terminally ill or permanently unconscious. Terminally ill in the legal sense means an illness from which one is unlikely to recover regardless of any possible treatment. So in this case, according to state law, the surrogates and the hospital personnel should have intubated. The treatment directive was not legally operative because this man was not terminally ill. They made a serious mistake, but it is understandable that they did. He was clear about his intentions and wrote them down. What was not grasped was the need to interpret living wills *not* simply from the perspective of what the person has written (the pure subjective standard, though in this case one could rightly argue that this is not what he really meant), but also from the perspective of the person's best interests.

But we need to look again at the idea that they should not have followed his treatment directive because the law says it was not operative. Do we want to make an absolute rule out of *that?* That would result in aggressive treatment for everyone not permanently unconscious or terminally ill. What if I write in my treatment directive that once my Alzheimer disease progresses to the point where I am no longer able to interact with my environment, I do not want to be hospitalized and intubated if I contract pneumonia? Then suppose I find myself in a situation where I am aphasic (unable to speak), confined to bed, and not only unable to recognize people but also unable to react with joy or with sadness to anything around me. I get pneumonia and they say it can be cured. The Alzheimer disease is not yet to the point where it is terminal in any immediate sense. Does this mean that since the state law says the treatment directive is not operative, I must be treated? No. As we have already seen, the Pennsylvania law (and this applies to many other state laws as well) is clear that this is all cumulative legislation. This may not be a statutorily enforceable operative treatment directive, but my surrogates and my physicians still may, and ought to, take it into consideration. They look at my wishes; they look at my best interests. They interpret. There is not any perfection in this; there is not any total control. There is seldom any way to be absolutely certain that my wishes will be followed unless I am able, here and now, to say what I want.

Emergency Blood

There is another case I often use to show the need for interpretation, though I am less sure about my conclusion here compared to the case we have just seen. A thirty-year-old man comes to the ER after a traffic accident that has caused a serious internal hemorrhage. He can not communicate. If he does not get blood immediately, he will die. The ER physicians think that if he is transfused and undergoes uncomplicated surgery, he has a very good chance of complete recovery. But he has a card in his wallet that reads, "I am a Jehovah's Witness; do not transfuse." His wife confirms his membership in the Witnesses and refuses to consent to a transfusion. The doctor has only a minute or two to decide. What ought to be done?

Note again that in Pennsylvania this is not an operative treatment directive. Even if the card in his pocket is properly signed and witnessed, which would make it a statutorily enforceable directive in this state, it is not operative because he is not terminally ill in the sense in which the law defines that term. Treatment will probably cure him. But we have seen that nonoperative living wills still ought to be and legally may be taken into consideration. Surely this is enough evidence of his wishes. What is the doctor to do?

Though I am hesitant to say this, I would probably support transfusion. My reasoning would not be the kind of vitalism that overrides patient wishes, though some might judge that in this case I am too close to the vitalism side of the spectrum discussed in chapter 1. Here it seems that there is a reasonable possibility (though perhaps a slight one) that the man would not choose *now* to reject the transfusion if he could state his wishes. That is, there is a chance that rejection would not be his contemporaneous decision were he able to make one. There are documented examples of similar cases in which Jehovah's Witnesses, when actually faced with this decision, chose to ignore their previously stated wishes and asked for transfusion. And this has happened in my own clinical experience. Impending death focuses the mind in new ways. And it is even possible, though unlikely, that the patient was never truly a believing Witness in the first place. The card may have been for him a way to fit into a family with strong beliefs. This is not a criticism of the faith or the moral courage of Jehovah's Witnesses. Catholics, after all, have abortions and use birth control. Circumstances change, and people change their minds accordingly.

It should be clear that if the Jehovah's Witness in this case were able *now* to state his preferences and he chose to refuse transfusion, knowing that death would (almost certainly) follow, it would then be morally outrageous and criminal assault and battery to transfuse him. For me, however, there is not enough evidence to be sure this would be his wish were he to know his present circumstances. I need more evidence. For example, if he previously had been in a similar circumstance and had said clearly that even though he might well die, he would not accept blood, there would be enough evidence to be virtually certain of what he would choose now. Or if the physician had been his longtime internist and if they had spoken together about this over a long period of time, so that the doctor really did know that he meant it, that would be enough evidence. But as it stands, in this emergency, I think I would support the transfusion.

What about the possibility of a criminal charge being laid? I very much doubt this would happen (district attorneys do not often bring charges against physicians who save lives), and if it did, given the flexibility always granted to physicians in emergency situations, the charge would almost certainly be dismissed or the physician acquitted. This is even more likely given the absence of an operative treatment directive. A civil suit is more likely. But if a transfusion were withheld, the physician might also be sued by the man's children, who might claim that their now-dead father had told them that he really was not a Jehovah's Witness but carried the card to keep peace with his wife. Which jury is easier to face, one hearing the grieving children of a man say that their father did not want to die or one hearing a perfectly healthy man charge you with saving his life? Theoretically, neither lawsuit should prevail.

Doctors' Orders and Charted Order Forms

Decisions made by the patient or a surrogate must be translated into doctors' orders. The treatment directive is not an order form. The mere fact that an advance directive is on the chart *means nothing* about what will actually be done until the patient's wishes, properly interpreted by surrogates in communication with physicians, become actual orders on the chart.

The easiest way to make this clear is to use the example of healthy people with living wills who are admitted to hospitals for the treatment of easily fixed medical problems. They should be resuscitated if something goes wrong and they arrest; they are not to be made DNR simply because they have a living will. Such would be another example of missing the needed interpretation. I have already noted that some people deliberately deny that they have an advance directive if they are hospitalized for a simple illness. If they should arrest during an appendectomy, for example, as a result of an anesthesia reaction, they *do* want CPR. It should not be necessary to hide advance directives. As long as hospital procedures make it clear that hospital staff follow the orders on the chart, and as long as there is proper discussion with the surrogate about how to interpret the living will (or with the competent patient about how to do so should she lose her ability to make decisions) and the resulting treatment decisions are entered into the orders section of the chart, advance directives will not be misused or misinterpreted.

Hospitals should design something similar to the Palliative Care Orders Form that was used in Pittsburgh's St. Francis Hospital before it closed in 2002. This is an *orders form*. Doctors fill it out and sign it, and they are supposed to do so after conversation with the patient or the surrogate. Palliative care forms are more sophisticated than simple code status because often the kinds of treatment chosen are more complex than what could be included in a code status, which is usually something simple such as "do not resuscitate," "comfort measures only," or "no aggressive treatment." If something goes wrong at two o'clock in the morning, the nurses and residents look to the Palliative Care Orders Form and follow it.

But there are sometimes problems even here. If the nurse discovers that the orders form is filled out in a way that contradicts the living will, this should be brought to the attention of the attending physician. If this does not resolve the issue, an ethics consultation is warranted. People write advance directives because they want their wishes to be honored. Interpreting them is not the same as ignoring them; indeed, it is the very opposite of ignoring them. And in order to make them effective, instructions must be entered in the chart and signed by the ordering physician (usually the attending physician).

PEOPLE WITHOUT SURROGATES

The law also wants to protect the rights of those who cannot make decisions about treatment, who have left no advance directives, and who have no one (no family, no close friends) who can serve as their surrogate. In order to do this, the law has tended to appoint a guardian and then expect that person to make decisions in accordance with the pure objective standard (the best interests standard), if there is no knowledge of the patient's wishes, or in accordance with other standards if, as is seldom the case, there is some knowledge of his or her wishes. But hospitals rightly hesitate to do this for a number of reasons. The most important is the problem of conflict of interest. An example might be a case in which paramedics bring a man, homeless and with no known family, to the ER. Doctors decide there is no hope for a meaningful recovery, but there is no one who can decide for the patient. If a guardian is to be proposed to the court, who should it be? Often hospitals propose their own social workers, but these people work for the hospital and are being asked to decide in the best interests of the patient, interests that may not coincide with the hospital's interests. Outside guardians are seldom available, and professional groups who offer this service naturally charge a fee—who will pay it?

For these reasons, some hospitals have added to their official policies on forgoing treatment a procedure to follow in such cases. At the University of Pittsburgh Medical Center, for example, a policy has been developed that some other Pittsburgh hospitals have adopted. If in such a case all the physicians agree that treatment cannot be of any benefit to the patient (it is clearly morally extraordinary), then a meeting of the ethics committee is called. For this purpose, the committee must consist of more than just the usual consultation team. It must include a specified number of members as well as representation from pastoral care, from the legal department, social work, and so on. If all unanimously agree with the doctors, then treatment is forgone. I think this is right, despite the fact that conflict of interest could still be a problem. We surely do not want to go to court on each of these cases. And in the present legal circumstances, as I have noted, guardianship is not likely to be a better solution. This approach has also been proposed by the New York State Task Force on Life and the Law (1993, 21–23).

THE PATIENT SELF-DETERMINATION ACT

In 1990 the federal government passed the Patient Self-Determination Act (PSDA), which went into effect on December 1, 1991. It is a rather simple law, though some law firms and some hospital associations seem to have embellished it and suggested added requirements to it that the law itself does not contain.

The federal law obliges all health care institutions that admit patients and accept federal funds (which means virtually all hospitals and nursing homes) to do the following three things. First, all admitted patients must be informed upon admission about state laws regarding patients' rights concerning choosing and rejecting treatment options. This should be done in writing, in easily read brochures handed to patients upon admission. Some states have a required or a suggested way to do this. It may be in legal jargon, and if it is, it is probably best to use it and then to add an explanation written by someone who writes for readers with less advanced reading skills.

Second, all admitted patients must be asked if they have an advance directive. The answer goes onto the patient's chart. If the answer is yes, the patient must be asked if he or she has a written copy of the directive on hand. If so, a copy goes into the patient's chart. If no, some attempt should be made to get a copy.

Third, the PSDA requires that all admitted patients be told about hospital policy concerning these issues. These policies should be available for patients to take and read. Though the PSDA does not mandate this, if a hospital's policy on these issues is not in line with the usual policies in the region, the hospital should inform admitted patients of what the unusual policy says and how it affects their rights to choose treatment. This might apply especially in any hospitals with so-called medical futility policies. These will be discussed in chapter 8.

Helping Patients Fill Out Advance Directives

All of this will lead patients to ask questions. They will want to know what a living will is and what a durable power of attorney or health care proxy is, and some may want to make one or both for themselves. Should the hospital help in this? There was some hesitation when the PSDA was originally passed, based on worry about conflict of interest, and some ethicists and hospital attorneys still recommend that hospital personnel not be involved in this process for their patients. In my opinion, this concern is overly cautious. Surely at the very least hospitals might suggest that patients choose surrogates to make decisions if they are unable to do so, thus aiding them in making a proxy directive. And many hospitals provide forms and offer some basic help to patients in designing simple treatment directives. More complicated directives, especially those requiring specific knowledge of the patient's present diagnosis and prognosis, should be made by the patient in dialogue with the physician. In any case, hospital personnel should not try to persuade patients in this. And it is better that it be discussed beforehand. It is also probably helpful if patients are given this information about advance directives again at discharge, though the law does not require this. Then they could look at it away from the traumatic context of the hospital, and they might be better prepared for the next admission.

Conclusion

I have devoted three chapters to the complicated question of who decides when treatment should be forgone. In general, capable patients may legally refuse virtually any treatment. This is, in the legal sense, the gold standard or ace of trump. But it does not apply to surrogate decision making. Surrogates may refuse only those treatments that are of little benefit or of great burden (best interests standard) or treatments that the patient, while capable of choosing, decided against (substituted judgment standard). The substituted judgment (subjective) standard should always be seen along with the best interests (objective) standard. Surrogates may (almost) never forgo treatment that is in the objective best interests of the patient, and advance treatment directives almost always require interpretation.

—❦ *Chapter 6* ❦—

Hydration and Nutrition

T HE ethical issue of withholding and withdrawing nutrition and hydration involves a specific application of the general principles developed in the previous chapters. There has been considerable controversy over whether or not nourishment and hydration can ever be omitted or discontinued for a dying or comatose patient, or for one who is in a persistent vegetative state.

The consensus in the United States is that nutrition and hydration may properly be forgone in some cases. The *Cruzan* decision of the Supreme Court upheld this general agreement (*Cruzan v. Director*, 1990), but there was considerable controversy along the way, and some ethicists and courts disagreed with the consensus as it emerged. In addition, over the past two years (2004 and 2005), debate over this issue has renewed, given impetus by the case of Terri Schiavo, which I introduced in chapter 4, and by an allocution delivered in March 2004 by Pope John Paul II, which, at least at face value, appears to require medical feeding for PVS patients.

A look at this issue, particularly at some of the related court cases and at the reinvigorated Catholic debate, will allow us to further study the interplay of the three pillars that form the basis of the current American consensus on forgoing treatment. In this chapter, I will argue that the Catholic tradition does *not* require hydration and nutrition for permanently unconscious patients, despite the claims of some that it does.

There are ethical questions as to when hydration and nutrition are morally ordinary and when they are morally extraordinary, and there are legal questions as to which means are always required in the law, which may be omitted and when, and who makes the decision. This issue is one that many hospitals and chronic care facilities face often, and it provides good test cases for the meaning of "ordinary" and "extraordinary" and for our care of the dying.

It is important to stress that the issue as it is usually framed is medical hydration and nutrition, involving the use of tubes inserted through the nose or directly into the abdomen, not ordinary food and water. Eating and drinking, food and water, have important symbolic meanings for humans (Carson 1989). They connote dining, human relationship, and, for Christians, the Eucharist. They must always be offered to patients who accept them. But this language is not appropriate in the context we are examining. For these reasons, it is better to use the proper words, "hydration" and "nutrition," rather than the words used for ordinary nourishment.

This does not mean, however, that health care providers are morally required to force food and water on those patients who, while physically capable of taking them by mouth, choose not to do so. Eating and drinking may indeed be morally extraordinary for some patients, even if the means are the usual ones and not medically assisted hydration and nutrition. In some cases, patients rightly determine that eating and drinking are not of any real benefit to them; they prolong the dying process and add to the patients' discomfort. The patients simply do not have the strength or the will to continue. In the words of the Vatican's Declaration on Euthanasia, a "correct judgment can be made regarding means, if the type of treatment, its degree of difficulty and danger, its expense, and the possibility of applying it are weighed against the results that can be expected, all this in the light of the sick person's condition and resources of body and spirit" (Congregation for the Doctrine of the Faith 1998, 653). The means may well be simple, but in some cases the patient's "resources of body and spirit" are such that even eating and drinking are morally extraordinary.

Thus, while food and water must always be *offered*, they need not always be *forced*. There are cases, of course, in which a person refuses to eat or drink as a result of some psychological illness or for some other purpose, as in a hunger strike. These cases present difficulties that cannot be judged a priori. In general, as we have seen, competent people can legally refuse all medical treatment, even life-sustaining treatment that is clearly morally ordinary from an objective perspective. In my experience, patients who refuse to eat even when their prognoses are good—they will probably recover from their condition—do so because of some psychological problem, often clinical depression. In these cases, it is better to try to find the cause of the problem than to automatically begin tube feeding. I remember one case in which it was simply a matter of turning on the television set in the patient's room and getting the right flavor of ice cream, a far better solution than a nasogastric tube. Nonetheless, there may be times when tube feeding is required against the wishes of an incompetent patient suffering from severe clinical depression. These cases will almost always concern patients with significant chances for meaningful recovery, however, not dying patients or those in terminal (irreversible) comas or persistent vegetative states.

The Persistent Vegetative State

The issue of forgoing nutrition and hydration often arises in the context of a persistent vegetative state. One of the earliest cases to be decided by the courts, that of Karen Ann Quinlan (*In re Quinlan*), involved a PVS patient. Paul Brophy and Mary Therese Schiavo, whose cases I will discuss in this chapter, were both in a PVS. And the papal allocution, to which I will return toward the end of this chapter, spoke of PVS patients. Thus is it helpful to introduce PVS before continuing. This is not to say, however, that the ethical and legal issues of hydration and nutrition are limited to patients in a

PVS. But since PVS patients can live for many years with feeding tubes, this condition has given rise to much of the debate.

There are a number of disorders of consciousness, to use the term of Joseph Fins (Fins 2005), and medicine is learning better to distinguish them. "Vegetative state" is a condition in which a person has lost the use of the cerebral cortex while the brain stem continues to function. I would prefer another term here, something other than "vegetative" because of the pejorative connotations of "vegetable," but this is the medical term used, and I will use it. The lower brain, or brain stem, controls certain bodily activities such as breathing, while the "higher brain," or cerebral cortex, controls the functions we usually think of when we think of human activity, such as thinking, emotion, and awareness of self and others.

A vegetative state is similar to but technically different from a coma. Both comatose patients and patients in PVS are completely unconscious and totally unaware of anything in the environment. But the coma victim is "asleep," that is, the eyes are closed, whereas the person in a PVS has sleep-wake cycles and is therefore at times biologically "awake," with eyes open. Comas do not last as long as vegetative states can; comatose patients die, become vegetative, or recover.

Because the brain stem continues to function, most PVS patients breathe without any medical support. Their eyes open and close and wander about. There are facial movements that can seem to be facial expressions. Their bodies move and there can be sounds like groans and sighs or other noises. None of these are in response to anything that goes on around them. These unconscious movements occur whether or not anyone is present. It is understandable that a loving family will interpret these movements and sounds as attempts at communication, as proof that their loved one is still aware of their presence, but, unfortunately, such a patient has lost the ability to do this. (The heavily edited tapes of Terri Schiavo that we saw so often on television, the purpose of which was to convince others that she was conscious, gave an appearance of awareness where there was none. Sadly, some who should have known better misdiagnosed her condition based on these tapes and other, similar reports.)

This kind of state is diagnosed as persistent or permanent after a period of time has passed. The term *persistent vegetative state* is generally used to mean one from which there is no reasonable hope of recovery to a state of even minimal awareness. But this is not always the meaning of *persistent*. Sometimes a distinction is made between a *persistent* and a *permanent* vegetative state (Mappes 2003). When this distinction is made, *persistent vegetative state* refers to the original diagnosis that a person is indeed in such a state and that it has persisted for a time, without implying that the patient can never emerge from it. Then *permanent vegetative state* becomes a prognosis that no recovery is likely (Mappes 2003, 124). Before it is made, this prognosis requires further observation and/or further tests.

An important 1994 article in the *New England Journal of Medicine* (Multi-Society Task Force 1994) describes recovery from a persistent vegetative state to at least a minimal level of consciousness, though not necessarily to functional capacity, as being as high as 52 percent (1572). Obviously this is not a permanent state of unconsciousness. In this article *persistent vegetative state* designates the condition after one month, with no implication of permanence (1499). Permanence is a prognosis made after further observation—three months post anoxia and six months post trauma, according to Fins, depending on the cause of the cerebral injury (Fins 2005, 22). This is based on the likelihood of recovery after this length of time. When such a distinction is made, it is possible that a patient can recover some awareness, even significant awareness and function after being in a persistent vegetative state, but this is not likely after this state has become permanent. Unfortunately, the acronym PVS is applied indiscriminately to both states, although the original term, *persistent vegetative state*, implied permanence and required a period of waiting before the term could be applied. The two different usages result in confusion.

I think it better to continue to use the term "persistent" and to wait before making this diagnosis until one can be reasonably sure that the state is indeed permanent. In my hospital experience, the distinction between "persistent" and "permanent" is not observed. *PVS* means persistent vegetative state, and it implies both the diagnosis of the condition and the prognosis of its permanence. This is the usual medical and bioethical usage. Beauchamp and Childress (2001), for example, use the term this way throughout their standard textbook, and I will use it that way here.

Proper diagnosis of "persistent-permanent vegetative state" is possible when it is based on laboratory studies and clinical observation, especially when this is supported by positron emission tomography (PET). With such tools, recovery can be virtually, and reliably, ruled out. A statement to this effect was made by the American Academy of Neurology (American Academy of Neurology 1989; Munsat, Stuart, and Cranford 1989). MRI (magnetic resonance imaging) and CT (computed tomography) scanning can also help by showing any structural damage.

Patients who are in a PVS are incapable of thinking. They are not aware of anything or anyone around them. They are not aware of themselves. They cannot dream. They cannot pray. They cannot recognize music or color or taste or touch. And they cannot experience pain or discomfort. This means that they cannot experience hunger or thirst even if their bodies lack food and water. This is a hard concept to grasp. If we are hungry or thirsty, we experience it; we want food and water. But PVS patients do not. They are entirely unaware of what is happening to them. In this life they are permanently beyond suffering, just as they are permanently beyond joy.

The American Academy of Neurology statement gives clear support to the withdrawal of nutrition and hydration from PVS patients. The academy also insists that PVS patients, despite their ability to breathe and open and move their eyes, are totally unconscious and cannot experience pain or suffering in any way. The withdrawal of nutrition and hydration does not, therefore, cause any sensation of dehydration or starvation.

One must be careful, however, to avoid being too quick to diagnose PVS and permanent coma. I have seen cases where these terms are used inaccurately. Good neurologists will want to be sure of the cause of the problem before deciding that a patient cannot recover from a coma. But we must not allow the possibility of misdiagnosis to cause us to ignore all diagnoses. As I noted in chapter 1, the only way to be absolutely sure to avoid all undertreatment, in the hope that a diagnosis is wrong and that the patient will recover, is to treat all illnesses aggressively regardless of diagnosis and prognosis, to do everything possible to preserve physical life. And this, as we have seen, is not required by the American ethical consensus or by Catholic tradition.

Legally, PVS and other forms of permanent coma do not fit the usual definitions of terminal illness. As we have seen in chapter 5, state laws usually define terminal conditions as those from which a person is likely to die in a short time (six months is often used) regardless of what treatments are applied. But PVS patients can live on for years, even for decades, with tube feedings and, usually, periodic antibiotics to treat infections. In another sense, however, permanent comas *are* terminal. The patient will die of this condition unless treatment is given. It is a "lethal" condition if not legally a "terminal" one.[1]

The *Brophy* Case

A court case that is particularly helpful in analyzing these issues is that of Paul Brophy, a Massachusetts firefighter (*Brophy v. New Eng. Sinai Hosp., Inc.*, 1986). Both Karen Ann Quinlan and Paul Brophy were diagnosed, correctly as far as anyone can tell, as being in a persistent vegetative state.[2] The difference between Quinlan and Brophy, however, was that Quinlan received ventilation and medical nutrition, whereas Brophy received only nutrition, which was provided by a feeding tube. (Many patients with PVS can breathe without mechanical assistance, since breathing is controlled by the brain stem, which is still functioning.) In the *Quinlan* case, the New Jersey court held that the ventilator might be removed and that generally speaking this should not be a court decision. Rather, a family member should be appointed guardian and given authority, in conjunction with any ethics committee the hospital might have, to turn off the ventilator ("In re Quinlan" 1982, 170). Most ethicists have applauded the *Quinlan* decision, and I agree. This kind of decision ought seldom to be in the courts, and the New Jersey Supreme Court made this clear when it overturned the superior court decision that had refused to allow Quinlan's father, Joseph, to discontinue ventilation. The New Jersey Supreme Court relied on Quinlan's right of privacy as a basis for her freedom from this kind of procedure (Meisel 1989, 98; 1995, 1:503–4). Quinlan actually lived for years after the ventilator was removed because nutrition and hydration were continued, but she never came out of her persistent vegetative state. The argument in this chapter is that nutrition might also have been removed, but this was not requested in Quinlan's case.

But what about Brophy? Here Judge David Kopelman of the Norfolk County Probate Court in Massachusetts refused to allow Brophy's wife, Patricia, to stop nourishment by the feeding tube. The court made a number of judgments that many ethicists have since criticized, though some have supported one or another of them.[3]

First, the court stated that even though Brophy had said over and over again that he would never want this kind of treatment, he had to have it anyway. Brophy had actually thrown away a commendation he received for saving a man from a burning car since the man had later died, and Brophy had judged his treatment to be useless. He also had commented to his wife that he never wanted to be like Karen Ann Quinlan.

Second, the court ruled that it would have been right not to insert the tube in the first place (in ethical terms, this meant the judge felt that this was "extraordinary" since it was clearly invasive), but that once the stoma, or opening, had been created and the tube inserted, the nourishment was a procedure of maintenance only (in ethical terms, the judge might have used the term "ordinary") and must be continued. That is, the judge insisted on a moral and legal difference between withholding and withdrawing treatment.

Finally, the judge stated that removing feeding is different from removing ventilation, since removing ventilation does not include necessarily the intent to terminate life, whereas removing nourishment does. In the ethical terminology we have already seen, he might have said that removing a ventilator is "allowing to die," whereas removing a feeding tube is active euthanasia or "direct" killing.

Four Questions

Was the judge correct in his opinions? In my judgment, and in that of most ethicists and jurists, the answer is no. There are four questions involved. Is stopping treatment different from not starting it? Is a feeding tube ethically different from a ventilator? Is withdrawing nutrition euthanasia, that is, is it killing as opposed to allowing to die? Who should make the decision to forgo or not to forgo treatment?

First, is there a difference between not doing a procedure in the first place (not creating a stoma and inserting the tube) and withdrawing a procedure that has been started (removing the tube and stopping nourishment)? The judge clearly thought so. With few exceptions, ethicists do not recognize that distinction as morally or legally relevant.[4] It is easy to see what would happen if we insisted on the difference. A person is brought to the emergency room, and the health care team cannot determine easily whether or not the patient can recover if resuscitation procedures are begun. So they begin them. The result is later found to be merely a prolongation of the dying process, not a treatment that will result in recovery to meaningful human living. If it is now wrong to stop what was started, medical professionals would be caught in an impossible ethical bind. Either they do not start treatment and fail to cure some patients or they start and then are required to continue useless measures for some patients. The Catholic tradition, with the distinctions we have discussed, has been able to avoid this bind. There is no moral difference between stopping and not starting. If the treatment is extraordinary, it is right to decide not to start it; it is also right to stop it once started. The American ethical and legal consensus has come to agree with this, and the *Cruzan* decision of the Supreme Court affirmed this consensus. The judge in *Brophy* was wrong.

Second, is a gastrostomy tube morally different from a ventilator? That is, in PVS and similar patients, is a gastrostomy tube an ordinary means of supplying nutrition and hydration while a ventilator is an extraordinary means of supplying air? There is some controversy about this among Catholic moralists, but it is clear that the main line of the Catholic tradition has argued that this kind of nourishment, along with intravenous feeding and other methods of nutrition and hydration, are indeed extraordinary in cases such as this. This distinction is not so much medical or technical as it is moral. Medical procedures that would be ordinary in some situations, where they might be reasonably expected to help, are clearly extraordinary, even unreasonable, in other cases, and the example of Paul Brophy is such a case. Medical feeding and hydration in this kind of situation are extraordinary. They are not the same as offering food and water to a starving or dehydrated person. Indeed, in cases in which nutrition and/or hydration are needed for patient comfort, they must always be given. Decades ago Jesuit moralist Gerald Kelly, accepted by all Catholic moralists as being consistent with official church teaching, clearly stated that artificial feeding may be discontinued (Kelly 1950).[5] This withdrawal is clearly permitted by Catholic medical ethics.

This answer to the second question gives us the answer to the third as well: Was the judge right in arguing that the intentionality of stopping feeding was "to kill," that is, in ethical terms, active euthanasia? In my judgment, and in that of most other moralists, including a strong majority of Catholic moral theologians, this was not active euthanasia, but was instead the stopping of an extraordinary and unreasonable means of preserving life. In cases like this, it is the disease that kills the patient, not the forgoing of treatment. Thus, the withdrawal of nutrition and hydration in such cases is permissible (indeed, since Brophy had clearly stated he did not want this type of treatment, its withdrawal is, in my opinion, morally required). But there is still controversy about this question, and I think that some of it results from confusion about the complex issue of intentionality that we considered in chapter 2. Families who withhold or withdraw feeding from permanently comatose loved ones do not intend their death in the sense of an end to be sought, even though they may well be relieved that death will bring peace and an end to a life in which no human action or experience is possible. And there is no reason to hold that the family's intention when forgoing feeding differs in any way from their intention in forgoing ventilation or other life-sustaining treatments. The Catholic tradition holds that in cases such as Brophy's, medically induced nutrition and hydration may be forgone.[6] And this proposal has become, with some disagreement still remaining, part of the American consensus about this issue.

It is interesting to note what finally happened to Paul Brophy. The Massachusetts Supreme Court overturned the decision of the probate court and ruled that the gastrostomy tube might legally be removed, though it refused to compel doctors to remove it. The tube was removed on October 15, 1986, and Brophy died on October 23, three and a half years after he had first lapsed into unconsciousness, and some two years after his wife had first asked that the gastrostomy nourishment be stopped ("Latest Word: In the Courts" 1986; "Latest Word: Brophy Dies" 1986). Most cases of this type have been similarly resolved, some more quickly, some not—for example, New Jersey's Nancy Jobes case (*In re Jobes*, 1987) Connecticut's Carol McConnell case (*McConnell v. Beverly Enters.*-

Conn., Inc., 1989), Pennsylvania's Jane Doe and Daniel Fiori cases (*In re Doe*, 1987; *In re Fiori*, 1996), Florida's Terri Schiavo case (*In re Guardianship of Schiavo*, 2003; *Bush v. Schiavo*, 2004; *Schiavo ex rel. Schindler v. Schiavo*, 2005), and a number of others.

The fourth question is who is best able to make the decision? As we saw in chapter 3, morally and legally, if the patient is competent, the patient decides. The Supreme Court's decision in *Cruzan* has upheld this. The question in cases like *Quinlan* and *Brophy* has to do with patients who are not able to decide. Now who makes the decision?

I dealt with this question in chapters 4 and 5 and need only make a few points here. In the *Quinlan* case, the court said that Quinlan's father, together with an ethics committee, if such existed at the hospital, should decide. This is the best approach. In the *Brophy* case, the probate court rejected the idea that his wife could decide. The Supreme Court of Massachusetts overruled the substance of the decision, deciding that the feeding tube might be removed, but did not rule, as in *Quinlan*, that the family should be the ones to decide. And in *Saikewicz*, a similar Massachusetts case, the court agreed that treatment could be stopped but explicitly rejected the New Jersey decision in *Quinlan* and insisted that the court was the only proper place to decide such issues (*Superintendent of Belchertown State Sch. v. Saikewicz*, 1977; Meisel 1989, 238–39; 1995, 1:237–38). The same conclusion was reached by a New York court in the so-called Brother Fox case (*In re Eichner*, 1979) but was later reversed (Meisel 1989, 244; 1995, 1:242). And in some cases in New Jersey, in which nursing home patients have been affected, involvement of the state ombudsman has been mandated (Meisel 1989, 252–54; 1995, 1:269–71).

Legally, therefore, the question of who decides is controverted. There does seem to be a general movement in Massachusetts, New York, New Jersey, and other states away from this unfortunate insistence on court or government action (Meisel 1989, 238–48; 1995, 1:239–46). Most ethicists, along with many jurists, would like to see a general acceptance of the *Quinlan* decision: In most cases, the decision ought to be left at the level of the family and the health care team, with the hospital's ethics committee as a possible resource. And in most jurisdictions, this is indeed the case.

CONSENSUS AND CONTROVERSY

Over the past several decades American courts have worked toward a general agreement that hydration and nutrition may be withheld and withdrawn from PVS and other, similar patients. The growing consensus accepts arguments from the Catholic tradition that medically induced nutrition and hydration may well be extraordinary means and that they may rightly be withheld or withdrawn. This consensus, as I have described it, is the approach taken by the 1983 report of the President's Commission for the Study of Ethical Problems in Medicine and Biomedical and Behavioral Research (1983, 90, 159–60, 196), by the New York State Task Force on Life and the Law (1992, 211–21) and by the Hastings Center in its 1987 *Guidelines* (1987, 59–62). The American Medical Association (1986, 2) advises doctors that artificial nutrition and hydration may be removed from patients who are near death and from those who are irreversibly comatose, provided the family or other surrogate concurs. Similar positions have been taken by the American Academy of Neurology (1989) and the American College of Physicians (1990).

But there has been and still is some significant debate among Catholic bishops and theologians (May 1998, 1999; O'Rourke 1999), much of which preceded the *Schiavo* case and the papal allocution. In New Jersey, for example, the state conference of Catholic bishops argued in the Jobes case that artificial nutrition must be maintained (*In re Jobes*, 1987). Yet in a similar case in Rhode Island, Bishop Louis Gelineau agreed that artificial nutrition could be stopped for a patient, Marsha Gray, in a persistent vegetative state. Oregon and Washington bishops issued a statement that supported the possibility of forgoing nutrition for permanently unconscious patients (Oregon and Washington Bishops 1991, 350), and so did Texas bishops (Texas Bishops 1990). Bishop John Liebrecht's statement on *Cruzan* also allows this (Liebrecht 1990). The Catholic Health Association of Wisconsin (1989) issued similar guidelines. But the U.S. Bishops' Pro-Life Committee (1992) issued a statement in 1992 that makes a strong presumption in favor of continuing to feed permanently comatose patients, a statement that was criticized by Kevin O'Rourke, a strong defender of the received Catholic tradition (O'Rourke and deBlois 1992).

The Pennsylvania Catholic bishops issued in 1991 a statement that seems to require hydration and nutrition for all or almost all PVS patients. Since the PVS patient is not terminally ill, they say, and since feeding tubes are providing a benefit by sustaining life with no burden to the patient, "the feeding . . . remains an ordinary means of sustaining life and should be continued" (Pennsylvania Bishops 1992, 548). These claims are precisely the ones I have argued the Catholic tradition rejects. Feeding tubes for PVS patients can be said to provide a benefit only by using that term as the Catholic tradition on ordinary and extraordinary means does not use it, as a medical term, not a moral one. There is no *human* benefit to these patients in keeping their bodies alive. Richard McCormick, one of the most influential Catholic moral theologians of the second half of the twentieth century, ends his article on the Pennsylvania bishops' statement this way:

> Let me conclude with a fanciful scenario. Imagine a 300-bed Catholic hospital with all beds supporting P.V.S. patients maintained for months, even years by gastrostomy tubes. Fanciful? Not if the guidelines of the Pennsylvania bishops are followed. Appalling? In my judgment, yes—not least of all because an observer of the scenario would eventually be led to ask: "Is it true that those who operate this facility actually believe in life after death?" (McCormick 1992, 214)

An unpublished document distributed to American dioceses in 1988 by the Pope John XXIII Medical-Moral Research and Education Center, titled "Feeding and Hydrating the Permanently Unconscious and Other Vulnerable Persons: A Report to the Congregation for the Doctrine of the Faith," requires hydration and nutrition for these patients.[7] But it includes criticisms, some of them rather scathing, by a number of Catholic moral theologians. Among these are rejections of the main conclusions by two "conservative" Catholic moral theologians. On theological grounds, Benedict Ashley correctly rejects the document's central argument that physical life can never be a burden and argues that the fight against euthanasia is better waged by holding to the Catholic tradition that permits the cessation of unwarranted treatment than by rejecting that tradition. Albert S. Moraczewski, of the Pope John XXIII Center, whose illness prevented him from chairing the drafting group, makes a series of statements that, on the basis of traditional Catholic moral theology, convincingly refute the main arguments of the document.

The *Ethical and Religious Directives for Catholic Health Care Services* includes a directive concerning medical nutrition and hydration that is helpful in resolving this controversy. Directive 58 and the introductory narrative to part 5 make it clear that hydration and nutrition for permanently unconscious patients cannot be said to be always obligatory on the basis of official Catholic teaching. The directive, which stands in clear contrast to those episcopal conferences that have claimed or at least implied that hydration and nutrition are obligatory, states: "There should be a presumption in favor of providing nutrition and hydration to all patients, including patients who require medically assisted nutrition and hydration, as long as this is of sufficient benefit to outweigh the burdens involved to the patient" (United States Conference of Catholic Bishops 2001).

For patients in a persistent vegetative state, there is no benefit in nutrition and hydration that can even remotely be considered a human benefit. In their commentary on the *Ethical and Religious Directives*, deBlois and O'Rourke state: "In theological terms, prolonging the life of persons in PVS does not seem to enhance their ability to strive for the purpose and goods of life" (deBlois and O'Rourke 1995, 27). It is interesting to note that the *Directives* do not require that the forgone nutrition be artificial. If seriously ill patients do not want to eat, and if eating is not of sufficient benefit to outweigh the burdens, this may be forgone. Patients with swallowing reflexes need not be force-fed any more than patients without them need be provided with medical nutrition and hydration.

Recent Catholic Controversy

Disagreement about hydration and nutrition for PVS patients has seen renewed vigor as a result of *Schiavo* and due to a formal talk given—partially given is more accurate, as I will explain—by Pope John Paul II on March 20, 2004 (John Paul II 2004).

Schiavo

There is no need to go into detail about the reaction coming from various Catholic bishops, priests, and theologians to the *Schiavo* case as it worked its way through the courts from 2003 to 2005. Some of it was in the context of the papal allocution, and I will consider the authority of that speech and some of the different interpretations given to it later in this section (see Cahill 2006, 124–32, for further statements and comments, on both *Schiavo* and the allocution). Catholics who commented on the case were just as likely to be misled by the media as were others, such as a number of politicians, who insisted that Terri Schiavo was not in a PVS. One Catholic bishop, for example, wrote a statement that pointed explicitly to the media as his source for claiming that "since she is still aware," withdrawing hydration and nutrition would cause her to suffer "an excruciatingly painful death" (Wuerl 2005). The statement of the Florida bishops asked for continued feeding until her condition was clarified. They rightly stated, "If Mrs. Schiavo's feeding tube were to be removed because the nutrition she receives is of no use to her, or because she is near death, or because it is unreasonably burdensome for her, her family, or caregivers, it could be seen as permissible." This is correct according to Catholic teaching, as we have seen. Unfortunately, the Florida bishops also said that the feeding tubes could be withdrawn "where that treatment itself is causing harm to the patient or is useless because the patient's death is imminent" (Florida Catholic Conference 2005). These two statements, while not flatly contradicting each other, stand in some tension. Treatments are morally extraordinary when their burdens outweigh their benefits, and this does not necessarily require that the treatment itself cause actual harm or that the patient's death be imminent.

This same claim, put even more strongly, that tube feeding is required unless a person's death is imminent, appears in other episcopal statements on *Schiavo* (Burke 2005; Morlino 2005) and in statements of other Catholic commentators (Mulligan 2005). As Thomas Shannon and James Walter (Shannon and Walter 2005a, 656–57) and Kevin O'Rourke (O'Rourke 2005, 549) point out, this requirement is simply not part of the Catholic tradition. To claim that treatment can be morally extraordinary only when a person's death is imminent, regardless of whether the treatment is given, is to give biological life itself an absolute value that supercedes all other values. This undercuts—indeed, in large measure it eliminates—the entire centuries-old Catholic distinction between ordinary and extraordinary means. It moves Catholic medical ethics toward a vitalism that it has until now correctly resisted.

The Papal Allocution

On March 20, 2004, Pope John Paul II talked to "400 participants in an international congress promoted by the World Federation of Catholic Medical Associations (FIAMC) and by the Pontifical Academy for Life" (Vatican Information Service 2004). In his allocution, the pope clearly stated that hydration and nutrition are morally ordinary treatment for PVS patients and that forgoing this treatment is "euthanasia by omission" (John Paul II 2004, 740). As should be clear from this chapter, this claim, in my judgment, is inconsistent with the received tradition of Catholic medical ethics. Because much attention has been paid to this talk, it is important to discuss its authority and how to understand it.

I will start with the question of the authority and importance of the talk. Catholic teaching distinguishes internal and external authority. Internal authority comes from the integrity of the arguments and their consistency with the rest of Catholic tradition on this and similar issues. From what has already been said, as well as from what I will note in this section when I suggest ways to interpret the talk, it would appear that the internal authority of the talk is not very high. It is not consistent with the rest of Catholic teaching on forgoing treatment and it does not, in my opinion, introduce any convincing new arguments as to why that teaching should be changed concerning nutrition for PVS patients.

External authority comes from the authority of the author of the document as well as from the way in which it is proclaimed. Papal documents are more authoritative in this sense than documents authored by individual bishops. Formal encyclical letters are more authoritative than more simple papal statements. Decrees from an ecumenical council, such as Trent or Vatican II, which have been approved by the pope and by all the gathered bishops, are generally seen as more authoritative than encyclicals, and so on. Thus the external authority of this talk is not very high. This is not an encyclical letter or a formal declaration but simply a talk Pope John Paul was asked to give to a meeting in Rome. In addition, there is significant doubt about the degree of papal involvement in the statement, because when the Holy Father was asked to give the talk, he was suffering from serious effects of Parkinson's disease. It is of course difficult to know exactly how much attention he was able to give to the allocution—the Vatican is understandably reluctant to speak publicly about a pope's health—but it is known that John Paul II was unable to finish giving the speech. It had to be finished by someone else, who read the document for him. In my judgment, and in that of others I have spoken with, it is possible that the Holy Father was unable to give any attention to the talk at all; it was simply something he was given to deliver at a meeting of physicians. In any case, the external authority of this talk is not high.

Nonetheless, because it was a papal address, a good deal of attention has been paid to it. I have seen a number of interpretations of this document—I will list four—some of which are careful and explicit, some less careful and implicit.

The first interpretation is that the talk does indeed mean what it seems to mean and that it marks a major and dangerous change in Catholic tradition. This is the interpretation of Thomas Shannon and James Walter (Shannon and Walter 2004, 2005a) and it is the one to which I subscribe. Shannon and Walter claim that the speech "seems to represent a significant departure from the Roman Catholic bioethical tradition" (Shannon and Walter 2004, 18). They worry that this has implications not only for PVS and feeding tubes, but for the wider tradition as well. And they point out a number of theoretical and practical problems, some of which I will return to later when I conclude this section.

The second interpretation, which seems the basis for a number of defenses of this position, is that the allocution applies only to PVS and (possibly, though not certainly) other, similar states, and that it applies only to feeding tubes and not to other procedures. Thus it does not imperil the tradition as a whole; it is a very limited application issue. This interpretation seems to me not to be carefully developed. There is no defended basis for making a moral distinction between feeding tubes, which are mandated, and ventilators, which are not. This seems to ignore the centuries-long requirement that Catholic moral theology has to be reasonable and coherent. Claiming that only feeding tubes are mandated, and that they are mandated only in PVS, introduces an incoherence into the tradition. If indeed it is morally mandatory to feed PVS patients for year after year with no human benefit—if this is an ordinary means of preserving their lives—then it is hard to see what could be called extraordinary. Perhaps some treatments that would themselves be enormously painful or overwhelmingly expensive might still fit the definition, but surely we could not continue to say that ventilators and dialysis are extraordinary while feeding tubes are ordinary. And we could not say that the fourth round of chemotherapy for a person with metastatic cancer is optional if that treatment had a small but nonetheless real chance of preserving life for a time. After all, the cancer patient could pray, could love, could think, could suffer—all humanly meaningful purposes of life. The PVS patient can do none of these things. If continuing biological life for the PVS patient is now said to be a human moral benefit that outweighs the costs and other burdens of the treatment, then surely any treatment that, without overwhelming cost or burden, prolongs the life of a conscious person, would have to be mandated as well. Thus this second interpretation, that this is a limited change applying only to feeding tubes for PVS patients, does not stand.

The third interpretation claims that the allocution does not change the tradition because although it applies "in principal," it still leaves room for individuals to decide that in their own situations feeding tubes for PVS patients are extraordinary and hence optional. This interpretation is proposed by Mark Repenshek and John Paul Slosar in response to one of the Shannon and Walter articles noted above (Repenshek and Slosar 2004). The authors agree that the tradition proposes a weighing of burdens and benefits. They correctly note that the tradition has applied to not just medical treatment but also other means of preserving life (Repenshek and Slosar 2004, 14), so that simply calling tube feeding "care" rather than "treatment" does not make it mandatory. They claim that, "given the origins of the principles . . . the address does not imply that medically assisted nutrition and hydration is obligatory for all patients in a PVS. As noted in the address itself, such care is only '*in principle* ordinary and proportionate, and *as such* morally obligatory.'" They go on to note that "the address does not state that an individual could not judge *for themselves* [*sic*] that medically assisted nutrition and hydration in the case of PVS would be disproportionate" (Repenshek and Slosar 2004, 15). If this interpretation is correct, it means that the allocution has no required application. It applies to few if any patients. At least it can be said not to apply by any who think it does not apply to themselves or to their unconscious loved ones. It is, rather, an "in-principle" exhortation to respect life. If this interpretation is correct, the allocution has little actual clinical impact. We should respectfully receive the exhortation but not think it changes what Catholic hospitals have been doing for decades.

The fourth interpretation is similar to the third. It claims that the allocution applies only to those in PVS for whom nonfeeding would cause suffering. The important section here from the allocution is this: "The administration of water and food . . . should be considered in principle ordinary and proportionate, and as such morally obligatory insofar as and until it is seen to have attained its proper finality, which in the present case consists in providing nourishment to the patient and alleviation of his suffering" (John Paul II, 2004, 739). Norman Ford, after quoting this passage from the allocution, states: "Hence it would no longer be morally necessary to provide MANH [medically assisted nutrition and hydration] if the patient is unable to assimilate it, or if it fails to alleviate suffering, or if it causes suffering" (Ford 2005, 3). Though Ford does not explicitly draw this conclusion, it would seem that, since PVS patient cannot suffer, feeding them never attains the finality of alleviating suffering, and so the allocution applies to absolutely no one. Here again, as for the previous interpretation, the allocution is really an exhortation to respect life rather than a decree that would change Catholic teaching and hospital policy.

Whether or not this talk will result in a change in official teaching is not yet clear. Some argue that the pope's speech means that the issue is settled and that Catholics (and, presumably, all people) are obliged to demand and to provide feeding tubes for all PVS patients (Latkovic 2005, 512; Furton 2005). Others remain faithful to Catholic tradition and insist that hydration and nutrition for PVS patients is morally extraordinary and hence optional (O'Rourke

2005; Eberl 2005; Shannon and Walter 2005a, 2005b, 2005c). Thus far there has not been any official change in Catholic hospital policy on the national level. The Catholic Health Association of the United States issued a brief "Statement on the March 20, 2004, Papal Allocution," noting that the "ethical, legal, clinical, and pastoral implications" of the allocution require careful consideration, and that "the guidance contained in the current *Ethical and Religious Directives for Catholic Health Care Services,* as interpreted by the diocesan bishop, remains in effect" (Catholic Health Association 2004).

REASONS AGAINST REQUIRING FEEDING FOR PERMANENTLY UNCONSCIOUS PERSONS

There are a number of reasons why traditional Catholic teaching permitting the nonuse of feeding tubes for PVS and similar patients ought not to change. I will list seven of them.

First, to do so would threaten the whole Catholic tradition of medical ethics. Why this is so should be clear by now.

Second, it would hurt real people. It would keep unconscious people unconscious, prevent their families from finding closure and moving on, and cause friction and distress among health care professionals. And in a bizarre way it might lead Catholic families to refuse treatment for patients who might recover rather than take the chance that they might lapse into a PVS. This is the possible result of interpretation two, described above. The new rule is said to apply only to PVS and to feeding tubes. There is still flexibility in other cases. So imagine a loved one has a bad stroke. While still in a coma, but not yet in technical PVS, she requires a ventilator. The doctors say she may recover awareness and even get better and go home, but it is more likely she will enter a PVS. Family members have been told that the allocution applies only to PVS and only to feeding tubes, so they believe that they can morally refuse the ventilator now. But if she goes into a PVS, they may be faced with twenty years of feeding tubes. So they refuse the vent. This may seem farfetched, but Joseph Fins has expressed this exact worry: "If an observant Catholic family were to follow Church teachings, they might be able to discontinue 'extraordinary' measures early in the patient's course when the prognosis was still unknown, but they might not be able to discontinue artificial nutrition and hydration later on, once it was clear that the patient would not make any progress from the vegetative state. The paradox is startling: A papal statement intended to promote life might have the unintended consequence of limiting the chance of recovery for some" (Fins 2005, 23). I have heard that such cases have actually occurred.

Third, the tradition ought not to change because the change would threaten Catholic hospitals. Despite the efforts of the Catholic Health Association to tell Catholic hospitals not to change anything, rumors are already circulating that some Catholic hospitals are refusing to honor advance directives. This may indeed be the case. People are starting to warn one another not to go to those hospitals. If Catholic hospitals were to be told not to honor advance directives about feeding tubes, as some writers are now insisting they do (Furton 2005), they would be required by federal law (the Patient Self-Determination Act, discussed in chapter 5) to tell all admitted patients this, which would severely threaten the hospitals. They and their doctors might even be open to criminal assault charges if they put tubes into patients whose directives refused them.

Fourth, the change suggests no belief in an afterlife: keep them here as long as possible. I quoted Richard McCormick's statement about this earlier in this chapter.

Fifth, surely such a change would be a violation of justice, spending so much on those who (1) can not benefit *and* (2) do not want the treatment in the first place.

Sixth, the change would lend support to the euthanasia movement. I will develop in detail in the next chapter why I am opposed to the legalization and practice of physician-assisted suicide and euthanasia. I think they are dangerous. But if I am forced to choose between being killed now and being stuck unconscious in a bed for twenty years with my family constantly in agony about it, I assure you, I will ask for euthanasia.

And finally, such a change would lend support to ethical relativism, that is, to the belief that there is no real basis for discovering right and wrong and that it is all a matter of personal, baseless opinion. When internal incoherence is introduced into Catholic medical ethics, it and the Church it comes from are relegated to the realm of the quaint. Isn't it interesting, people think, that the Jehovah's Witnesses won't take blood and the Amish drive buggies and the Catholics feed the permanently unconscious. Who knows what's right? It's all a matter of opinion. This danger is increased when Catholic moral theology moves in the direction of a decreed or posited (we used to say one thing, but now the Vatican has spoken so we say another instead) rather than a discovered body of knowledge (we know what is right and wrong because we can discover it using reason and experience to examine the nature and purpose of the human person as creature of God). Thus one of the last traditions of ethics (perhaps *the* last one) actually claiming to be reasonable and coherent and based in human purpose becomes just another contribution to contemporary ethical chaos, reduced to an arcane subject for study in graduate school.

Medically Futile?

One further related issue is the question of whether artificial nutrition might be removed from a permanently comatose patient against the wishes of the family or other surrogate. Currently, it is unwise and probably illegal to do so. The consensus as it has emerged thus far in the United States considers decisions such as these not medical ones in the strict sense, but value decisions or "quality of life" decisions. That is, no medical decision can be made that hydration and nutrition (as well as ventilation and other similar modalities) are medically futile in cases such as *Quinlan, Brophy,* and *Schiavo.* I agree with the approach that insists that such treatment cannot be called medically futile in the strict sense, such that physicians might unilaterally decide to forgo it. I will return to the issue of medical futility in chapter 8.

"STARVATION AND DEHYDRATION"?

When a person has irreversibly lost consciousness, there is no possibility that he or she will experience any of the effects of malnutrition or dehydration. But the ethical issue of forgoing hydration and nutrition is not limited to those in this condition. It can be morally extraordinary to use feeding tubes in other patients as well, as long as the principles for determining this are properly applied. Thus the question arises as to whether hydration and, perhaps, nutrition are always required as comfort measures for conscious patients. It seems clear that for very sick and dying patients the effects of dehydration are often actually benign (Printz 1989; Miller and Meier 1998). There is less fluid to cause breathing problems. Whatever discomfort there is can probably be alleviated by "maintaining moisture in the mouth with water, ice chips, or various forms of artificial saliva" (Billings 1985, 809). There is even medical evidence to suggest that tube feeding may be contraindicated, that is, inadvisable, in patients with advanced dementia who are not near death, as its burdens often outweigh its benefits in such cases (Gillick 2000). According to one study, tube feeding does not provide comfort and does not even significantly prolong patients' lives (Finucane, Christmas, and Travis 1999), and it may be right, therefore, to forgo it for patients with advanced dementia. The debate on this question is now underway (Burke 2001b; Kahlenborn 2001; Burke 2001a).

Terms such as "starvation" and "dehydration," while in one sense technically accurate, include implications that are almost never valid in the kinds of cases we have been considering. Clearly, if hydration and nutrition are necessary for the patient's comfort, they must always be used. But usually, in cases like these, they are not necessary for comfort. Rather, they serve only to prolong the patient's dying process and may in fact add discomforts of their own. Thus they are morally extraordinary and may rightly be withheld or withdrawn.

DETERMINATION OF DEATH

PVS patients and the permanently comatose are not dead by current U.S. legal standards. The Uniform Definition of Death Act (UDDA) makes it clear that death is the irreversible cessation of all cardiopulmonary function or, in the presence of ventilators that keep that function going, the irreversible cessation of all brain function, including that of the brain stem. Brain function is usually interpreted as integrating brain function—random electric events are not signals of life (Meisel 1989, 134; 1995, 1:625). All fifty states have accepted brain death as meaning, in the legal sense, that a person has died (Meisel 1995, 1:625). PVS patients have not lost function of the brain stem, which means that many continue to breathe on their own. In this chapter, therefore, I have spoken of living but lethally ill people, patients who will, unless morally extraordinary means are used to keep them alive, inevitably die of their condition.

BRAIN DEATH

Treatment is not "forgone" for the dead. No treatment can be given to the dead body of what once was a human being. Only the respect owed to corpses is proper. But there has been some development since the 1970s regarding how to determine that death has occurred. Prior to the use of mechanical ventilators that can keep the heart beating by providing it oxygen through the lungs, the determination of death was relatively simple, at least in theory. When a person stopped breathing, death was declared. There were in fact a considerable number of cases in which people in comas were thought to be dead and were buried alive. Devices were sometimes used to ensure that such people could signal were they to wake up in such a dire circumstance, but in theory the issue was easy enough. No breathing and no heartbeat meant that death had occurred. But with ventilators that changed, creating the issue of "brain death."

Brain death, according to the UDDA, is not different from any other kind of death. It is death pure and simple. It is arguably unfortunate that the term is used, because many think it means a different kind of death, an earlier death or even a preventable death. I think it is better, for example, when doctors must tell families that brain death has occurred, for them to say simply that the patient has died rather than to say that the patient is "brain dead." Of course, if the family wants to know the details, or has been involved in the process of the diagnosis, physicians have to be clear about what has happened.

Brain death refers to criteria used to determine that a person has indeed died when the usual criteria for determining this event (cessation of breathing and heartbeat) are not available because heart and lung function are being forced by machines. But no one who is declared "brain dead" would have been thought to be alive before the criteria and the machines that necessitated them were invented. Total brain death means virtually instant cessation of cardiac and pulmonary function in the absence of machines. Both the higher brain, the neocortex, and the lower brain and brain stem are dead. The person is dead. Heart and lungs may be forced to work, but this does not mean that human life of any sort continues. This definition is now almost universally accepted. Continued treatment of the brain dead is treatment, in effect, of a cadaver and is thus contrary to the standard of medical care. It is, in the meaning I will give to the term in chapter 8, medically futile.

Some controversy remains about how to respond to people who, for religious reasons, reject the notion of brain death and insist that the hearts and lungs of such people be forced to continue to function in the body, arguing that the person is alive. The most common judgment made here, one that I accept, is that religion cannot legitimately reject a medical fact and that brain death is indeed a medical fact and not a question of faith or personal philosophy. Death is an ontological state and not, as such, a social construct (though there is much that we socially construct about the process and meaning of dying and death).[8] People who are dead cannot properly be claimed to be alive. No medical treatment may be given to the dead. Those who believe that patient and family autonomy should always prevail in such cases and those who reject brain-death criteria dissent from this opinion. But the prevailing opinion, one held by a majority of ethicists and physicians, is that brain death is a medical determination that cannot be denied on other bases. At the very least, anyone insisting on ongoing treatment for the brain dead, that is, for dead people, should be asked to bear the total cost.

A second controversial issue concerns the determination of the status of people in irreversible comas and persistent vegetative states, those whose higher or neocortical brain functions have permanently stopped. As we have seen, these patients are not brain dead because their brain stems continue to function, but they have irreversibly lost all higher brain function. They are "vegetative" and will remain so, but their hearts and lungs will continue to function, usually without mechanical ventilation. In this chapter, I have discussed the ethical and legal issues concerned with forgoing medical nutrition and hydration in such cases, but these issues would be moot if we were to declare these patients dead. Some argue that this is precisely what we should do (Meisel 1989, 134–35; 1995, 1:627–30).

I believe that there is a legitimate theological argument for this approach, though I am not fully convinced.[9] It is clear, however, that society is not willing to claim that breathing bodies may be dead, to bury breathing corpses. In addition, there is a serious danger of backlash against organ transplantation, especially because it is mainly transplant specialists who are proposing that higher brain death be sufficient for declaring a person dead (Meisel 1995, 1:627). This context, harvesting cadaver organs, is a bad one in which to make this kind of decision. This is also true of the proposal to declare anencephalic infants to be brain-absent and therefore dead.

For now, only total brain death, including death of the brain stem, should be considered in declaring the patient dead. Total brain death simply introduces a new set of criteria for determining the same moment of death. But neocortical criteria, according to which the irreversibly comatose would be declared dead, would indeed push death earlier: Patients who, decades ago, would have been thought to be alive would now be said to have died. Physicians would have to intervene to stop the heart from beating and the lungs from breathing. Society is not ready for this and probably need never accept it. With the sensitive forgoing of treatment, patients in irreversible comas can be allowed to die. They need not be declared already dead.

One final argument supports this position. Decisions to forgo medical treatment for the living need not be traumatic, but neither should they be automatic. Declaring a person to have died allows an easy escape from what should be a decision requiring serious thought. Ethics should offer comfort and relief from false guilt and fear, but it should not adopt moral or legal shortcuts to turn important decisions into thoughtless ones. Comatose patients should not be declared dead; brain-dead patients have indeed died.

Notes

1. PVS patients are in fact dying; they are dying from the brain injury that makes it impossible for them to eat and drink, just as patients with end-stage lung disease are dying because their disease makes it impossible for them to breathe. Medically induced ventilation can keep breathing for

them, but they are still said to be dying patients, and if the ventilator is withdrawn, they die from the disease, not from the withdrawal of the ventilator. The same is true for patients in irreversible coma or PVS. They are dying of a disease that will kill them unless these morally extraordinary means are used to keep them alive. As another example, the cause of death in patients with end-stage heart disease is the disease, not the forgoing of a heart transplant. If this analysis were not true, forgoing extraordinary means of treatment would always be the cause of death and thus would be a direct killing. As we have seen, however, this is not the case, according to either U.S. law or Catholic medical ethics.

2. The court in *Quinlan* used the word "comatose" ("In re Quinlan" 1982, 170), and the two terms are often not properly distinguished.

3. On the *Brophy* case, see Annas 1986; Paris 1986; Bresnahan and Drane 1986; and Rothenberg 1986. For an opinion, given at the trial, insisting that the treatment be maintained, see Derr 1986.

4. I know of no secular ethicist who insists on the moral relevance of this distinction. I have heard religious leaders insist on such a distinction, and the Orthodox Jewish tradition has claimed such a relevance (Bone et al. 1990). For a different interpretation of the Jewish position, see Feldman 1986, 91–96; Dorff 2000, 348–54; and Mackler 2003, 97–98.

5. For citations in context by contemporary authors who are arguing the issue, see Paris 1986; Flynn 1990, 79; and McCormick and Paris 1987, 358. Gerald Kelly says that artificial means such as oxygen and intravenous feeding "not only need not but should not be used, once the coma is reasonably diagnosed as terminal" (Kelly 1950, 220). Some argument might remain about what is meant here by the word "terminal," but it is most likely, given the rest of Kelly's argument about benefit and burden, that what we now call "irreversible coma" and "persistent vegetative state" would fit. In this article, Kelly argues that these means are "ordinary" but "useless" and therefore optional, thus adding a confusing distinction that is not necessary if "ordinary" and "extraordinary" are considered as moral rather than medical terms, as I have proposed, and as is more in consonance with the development of the distinction in Catholic medical ethics. Kelly's later use of these terms clears up his confusion here (Kelly 1958, 129).

6. A particularly helpful brief review of the issues from the Catholic perspective is O'Rourke 1989. Another source, often cited, is the doctoral

dissertation by Daniel A. Cronin, later bishop of Fall River, Massachusetts, who supports the position that nutrition and hydration are not mandatory (Cronin 1958). McCartney (1986) gives a list of key citations from Catholic authors recognized as orthodox. Shannon and Walter (1988) supply an excellent analysis of the issues.

7. See also McHugh 1989 and May et al. 1987. This last is a summary of the report sent to the Congregation for the Doctrine of the Faith.

8. I do not intend to enter into the theoretical difficulties involved in the relationship among definition of death, criteria for determining death, and tests used to assure that the criteria are met in individual cases. Recent scholarship has noted these problems. From a theoretical perspective, the definitions and criteria claimed to support the UDDA are doubtless flawed. From a practical perspective, however, tests used to assure that total brain death has occurred are, in my judgment, when properly applied, sufficient to assure that the patient is indeed dead. For a particularly insightful exploration of these issues, see Chiong 2005.

9. See Janssens 1983. For my analysis of this argument, see Kelly 1988.

—☙ *Chapter 7* ❧—

Physician-Assisted Suicide
and Euthanasia

WE have seen that the American consensus on forgoing treatment has as one of its ethical bases the claim that there is a difference between killing terminally ill patients and allowing them to die of their underlying condition. The general agreement has been that while it is often right to withhold or withdraw medical treatment that would prolong the lives of dying people, it is not right to kill them or to help them to kill themselves.

There have always been, of course, those who disagree with this position. But only recently have we seen major turmoil in the United States about the ethics and about the law concerning euthanasia or physician-assisted suicide. There were states that did not have laws forbidding assisting suicide, and there were states that did (and still do), but to my knowledge until 1996 no cases had been decided concerning the constitutionality of such laws. Prior to this, there had been no real legal attack on what I have called the second pillar of the consensus.

RECENT LEGAL DECISIONS

In 1996 two important court decisions reached conclusions opposed to the general legal consensus about active euthanasia and physician-assisted suicide. And then, in June 1997, the U.S. Supreme Court reversed those decisions, returning the legal status to what it had been, but in doing so underlining the possibility that states may indeed proceed to pass laws legalizing PAS and, presumably, active euthanasia.

The United States Court of Appeals for the Ninth Circuit (covering Washington, Oregon, California, Alaska, and four other western states) and the U.S. Court of Appeals for the Second Circuit (New York, Connecticut, and Vermont) both decided in 1996 that certain state laws (those of Washington and of New York) forbidding physician-assisted suicide were unconstitutional (Meisel 2003, 479–93). Though neither of these decisions affected practice in other jurisdictions, and even in these states the practical effect was minimal as everyone waited for the anticipated Supreme Court appeals, there was for a time a real worry (or hope, depending on one's viewpoint) that all state laws forbidding PAS might be found unconstitutional.

The Ninth Circuit claimed that there is a constitutional right to choose the time and manner of one's own death that extends at least to terminally ill people, so that they may ask physicians to help them commit suicide (*Compassion in Dying v. Washington,* 1996). It appeals to the *Casey* abortion decision (*Planned Parenthood v. Casey,* 1992) and to *Cruzan v. Director* (1990) as supports for a liberty interest that is, or approaches the status of, a fundamental right to choose how and when to die. Laws making this illegal are thus unconstitutional (Meisel 2003, 479–88).

The Second Circuit argued more narrowly that the equal protection clause of the Fourteenth Amendment does not permit states at the same time to let terminally ill people choose to withdraw life-sustaining treatment, and thus die when and how they wish, *and* to forbid terminally ill people from asking doctors to help them kill themselves (*Quill v. Vacco,* 1996; Meisel 2003, 488–93). This, said the Second Circuit, illegally discriminates against those unfortunate enough to be dying and not on forgoable life-support. These people were not equally protected under the law. Both circuit courts claimed that the long-held distinction between killing and letting die is a false one. The Second Circuit cited Justice Scalia's minority opinion in *Cruzan* equating refusal of treatment with suicide as one of its bases for this judgment (Annas 1996, 187).

The Ninth Circuit decision includes bad history and bad analysis (Schneider 1997; Kamisar 1996). The court did not even take the time to understand the meaning of some of the ethical terms it was using. For example, it seems to have equated the distinction between withholding and withdrawing treatment with that between commission and omission, or active and passive euthanasia. As we saw in detail in chapter 2, withholding and withdrawing are *both* permitted as "passive euthanasia," a term, I repeat here, that is confusing and probably ought to be avoided. Withholding and withdrawing are both the "nondoing" of treatment and may well be right. The Second Circuit decision was better argued but still ultimately flawed. Despite Scalia's opinion, refusal of treatment is *not*, as we have seen, the same as suicide. And there are other reasons as well for rejecting the decisions of both circuit courts that I will give later in this chapter.

In June 1997, the U.S. Supreme Court reversed the decisions of both circuit courts (Meisel 2003, 493–510). It held, against the Ninth Circuit, that there is no constitutional right to choose when and how one dies, and it rejected the argument of the Second Circuit that there is no difference between forgoing life support and suicide, holding that it is not contrary to the equal protection clause of the Fourteenth Amendment to allow withdrawal of life support but to forbid assisting self-killing and euthanasia. Thus the Supreme Court stated that the Washington and New York laws forbidding assisted suicide are constitutional or, to be more precise, not unconstitutional on the grounds claimed by the circuit courts. We are thus back to where we were. States may pass laws forbidding euthanasia and forbidding assisting suicide. States need not pass such laws, of course. They may have no laws at all. Or they may specifically permit these practices, as Oregon has done for PAS.

The 1994 Oregon referendum and the subsequent law (Oregon Death with Dignity 1998) explicitly permitting physician-assisted suicide was not rejected by the Supreme Court's decision. Another federal court decision rejected it as unconstitutional, but the Supreme Court overturned that decision. In November 1997, another referendum in Oregon, which would have reversed the first referendum and thus made PAS again illegal in the state, failed by a vote of sixty to forty percent. Various attempts by federal and local initiatives, including rulings that using drugs for suicide would violate federal laws, also failed (Meisel 2003, 43–45), and the Supreme Court ruled in January 2006 against the attempt by the Bush administration to criminalize this use of drugs (Baron 2006). Thus PAS is now legal in Oregon.

In sum, though we are legally back where we were, much has been legally clarified, and the next battleground will be state legislatures. Their decisions are not easy to predict. After the decision in Oregon, many thought that other states would soon legalize PAS. But to date this has not happened. Oregon is alone. Indeed, some other states have passed laws forbidding PAS or have strengthened previously existing laws against the practice. As of 1999, thirty-seven states had laws specifically forbidding assisting at suicide, eight forbade it by common law or case precedent, and four were unclear (Doerflinger 1999).

This chapter is divided into three main sections. In the first I present a brief sketch of the definitions and distinctions necessary for understanding the issue. In the second I offer what I think are proper alternatives to PAS. And in the third I present a brief chronology of my own changing judgments on the question of whether PAS and euthanasia are morally right and ought to be legal.

Definitions and Distinctions

Physician-assisted suicide is generally understood to mean action by a licensed physician that provides to a legally competent person some means to use in committing suicide. Though it is not formally part of the definition, the context of the person's terminal illness is often assumed and has been part of the prerequisite conditions in all proposed laws thus far, as well as in the two decisions by the U.S. circuit courts. But this is not a formal part of the definition of physician-assisted suicide as such, since physicians might be permitted to offer such aid to those who wish to kill themselves for other reasons. In fact, many advocates include conditions that are not terminal in the sense the law commonly gives to that term, that is, a condition that will probably cause death within six months regardless of what treatments are applied. PAS is different from the withholding or withdrawal of life-sustaining treatment, on the one hand, and from the actual killing of the patient by the doctor (physician-administered euthanasia), on the other. The former action (withholding or withdrawal), as we have seen, is legal and recognized as ethically right by both the American ethical consensus and official Catholic teaching. The latter (active euthanasia) is forbidden as criminal homicide in all fifty states, and the recent court decisions do not address it directly, though, as I point out later, once we allow PAS we will almost of necessity have to allow active euthanasia in at least some cases.

A distinction is often made among voluntary, nonvoluntary, and involuntary euthanasia. *Voluntary euthanasia* is the killing of a person at that person's request. *Nonvoluntary euthanasia* is a killing in the absence of such a request and is usually proposed and debated in the context of incompetent people. *Involuntary euthanasia* is a killing of a person who explicitly rejects the offer. Physician-assisted suicide in the strict sense presupposes a voluntary act, as it is the patient who consumes the drug. Pressures that reduce the voluntary nature of the act might be brought to bear in order to convince people to accept the offer and take the drug. Similarly, less-than-competent people might be allowed to choose to kill themselves and then might be given lethal drugs. These two reductions in voluntariness are admittedly also possibilities when patients must decide whether to accept or forgo life-sustaining treatment.

Alternatives to Physician-Assisted Suicide

There are two humane and morally proper alternatives to PAS that are supported by the present consensus, along with a number of inhumane alternatives that, unfortunately, often occur. The inhumane alternatives to PAS include abandonment of patients to their own devices, refusal to care for them because their insurance is insufficient, inadequate pain management, and paternalistic insistence, against their wishes, on aggressive (morally extraordinary) life-sustaining treatment.

The two humane, legal, and morally proper alternatives are, first, the ethically right and legal forgoing of life-sustaining treatment and, second, proper pain management. I am convinced that if we were better at these than we are, we would reduce the perceived need for helping patients kill themselves, though we would not eliminate it altogether. As we saw in chapter 2, the process of dying inevitably brings with it what James Walter calls "agent narrative suffering," as distinguished from the "neurophysiological suffering" that pain relief can eliminate (Walter 2002, 6). To eliminate the existential anxiety that comes to so many of us as we die, and to eliminate the loss of bodily and mental control that accompanies dying, will doubtless remain reasons for requesting euthanasia and PAS. I have already noted, however, that even these factors can be alleviated with the care and compassion of health care providers, family, and others.

The Ethics of Assisted Suicide and Euthanasia

Even with the proper forgoing of treatment and proper pain control, there remain some reasons for physician-assisted suicide and euthanasia. What, after all, is the difference between giving dying people enough sedation to keep them unconscious until they die and simply killing them now or helping them to kill themselves while they still can? Why not just get it over with? Why maintain this antiquated notion that killing and allowing to die are ethically different?

We need to return to the ethical reasons for the second pillar of the consensus, the claim that there is a moral difference, and that there ought to be a legal difference, between killing and allowing to die. To get at these reasons, I will trace my own moral journey on this issue. I hope this will not be totally idiosyncratic and will help in an understanding of the claims made and the justifications given for them. My own moral judgment on this issue has gone through four stages, and I will use this as a framework.

Stage One

When I was in college, and during my early graduate school work, I was convinced that the reasons proposed by the received tradition of Catholic ethics for concluding that the direct killing of innocent people is absolutely wrong were valid. Basically, two reasons are given. First, it is argued that God keeps to God's self the right to kill the innocent, giving to humans only the right to kill the guilty and the right, sometimes, to allow the innocent to die. Second, it is argued that such killing of the innocent is an intrinsically evil or intrinsically wrong action, apart from intention, circumstances, and consequences. In this first stage I accepted these reasons as valid, and thus I held that euthanasia (and PAS, which was not really an issue then) was always wrong and ought to be illegal.

Stage Two

When I was working on my doctoral dissertation on the history and method of Catholic medical ethics (Kelly 1979), I became convinced that neither of the two reasons cited above worked. I developed these issues at length in my earlier book (Kelly 2004), and it is enough here to say that the first reason, that God keeps for himself the right to kill the innocent, turns out to depend on the second reason, the one about intrinsically evil acts. I did not think, and still do not think, that one can make valid ethical judgments based solely on acts themselves apart from human circumstances, intentions, and consequences. I accepted the arguments proposed by Daniel Maguire (1974) and concluded that euthanasia was sometimes morally right and that it ought to be legal as well.

Stage Three

In 1981, when I began teaching at Duquesne University and working on ethics committees in Pittsburgh area hospitals, this experience, and the reading I did around the issue, began to worry me. I became more aware of what I perceived to be the social consequences of the practice of euthanasia and more concerned about slippery-slope social results. So in *Critical Care Ethics* (Kelly 1991), I argued that although euthanasia might be morally right at least some of the time, it should not be legalized. My reasons, which I still think are valid, include the following.

First, any increase in the number of exceptions to the general principle against killing makes other exceptions easier. Our nation has decided that killing is legally permitted in properly declared wars, in court-ordered capital punishment, in abortion, in self-defense, and in some circumstances in defense of private property attacked criminally. Active euthanasia is not the same kind of killing as these others, but to permit it legally would add an additional exception to the law forbidding killing. This first reason is not convincing to everyone because of the difference between euthanasia and PAS and other kinds of legal killing. But I am convinced there is simply too much violence, and for me, PAS remains a violence.

Second, it would be very difficult, if not impossible, to hold the line at physician-assisted suicide and resist moving to voluntary and to nonvoluntary active euthanasia (New York State Task Force 1994, 144–45). This much is clear to me: If one accepts PAS, one must accept logically, and will have to accept legally, some kinds of euthanasia, certainly voluntary and probably nonvoluntary. I do not mean by this that I think that euthanasia advocates really want to do away with the old and the infirm. Far from it. Most are caring physicians and ethicists dedicated to helping the dying and alleviating suffering. But I do not see any valid moral reason for refusing a merciful death simply because a patient is not able, here and now, to ask for such a death or to do it unaided. Though laws might at first limit the practice to PAS, it would be hard to draw the line there, since one might logically insist that those incapable of choosing and of killing themselves should also have the right to be freed of the dying process. Surely, if we cross the line to allow physicians to provide lethal drugs to help in the suicide of a dying patient, we owe similar help to those competent, dying people unable to kill themselves—a quadriplegic requiring assistance to take the pills, for example. In this case, the action would technically be euthanasia, since the physician would have to put the pills in the patient's mouth. And if this is done, there is surely good reason to move toward euthanasia by injection instead, since lethal agents can be better introduced that way.

And what about those who asked for euthanasia in documents they wrote after they were diagnosed with a terminal illness? These people want to live on until they can no longer function humanly, so they ask that the drug be administered to them, not now when they still have reasons for living and can take it themselves, but later, when they are no longer able to interact. Surely these people have greater reason to have their lives ended than do those who wish to take the pills while they are still able. And this is clearly a case of euthanasia by previous directive. I think it is still voluntary euthanasia, but it is less immediately clear what the person would want now.

What about those who request euthanasia in an advance directive written before any specific diagnosis? If they suffer a sudden trauma that makes them permanently unconscious, should we refuse to honor that directive simply because they never had the chance to ask for drugs and take them themselves? This will open up the problems of interpretation I discussed in chapters 4 and 5.

And what about those who have never been able to ask for this help, such as children and those with a lifelong severe mental illness? We will certainly have to allow loving families to request that their dying loved ones be killed, or "euthanized," just as we now allow them to request the forgoing of treatment. It makes no sense *not* to do that.

And finally, what about a person who is not terminally ill in the strict sense but is diagnosed with a long-term chronic illness such as Lou Gehrig's disease (ALS)? What reason do we have to refuse "aid-in-dying" to such a person? Though perhaps we *can* hold the line at terminally ill or permanently unconscious people, what logical reason would we have for doing so? Medication can eliminate pain in the dying patient, but it will not help the quadriplegic walk again. It does not allow people with long-term progressive illnesses to escape the limitations those illnesses bring. So in some ways there is *greater* reason to help nondying people commit suicide or to kill them when they ask us (active euthanasia) than there is to do this for those whose deaths are imminent.

It is important to note that there is reason to think that once we legalize PAS, we will be required to legalize euthanasia for at least some of the categories of people I have described. It is likely contrary to the equal protection clause of the Fourteenth Amendment to limit such help to conscious people. The Supreme Court overturned the decision of the Second Circuit Court of Appeals on PAS, but it did not repeal the Fourteenth Amendment. Rather, it said that there is a relevant difference between forgoing treatment and PAS. It does not seem that there is a relevant difference among the kinds of patients I have described. At some point someone in Oregon will argue that the state law there is unconstitution because it unjustly discriminates in favor of people currently ab to ask for and consume the lethal drugs and against those wh annot. The Supreme Court may well have to rule that since son has permitted PAS, it must permit active euthanasia as

A great deal of controversy has arisen conce g evidence from The Netherlands on this question. For some though euthanasia remained technically illegal, there was an agreement that physicians who practiced it would not be prosecuted as long as they followed certain criteria (euthanasia under these criteria is now technically legal in The Netherlands). One of these criteria is that the person to be killed must ask to die. But there is clear evidence, based on the Dutch government's own 1991 Remmelink Report, that a significant number of those killed—infants, children, and the unconscious, for example—do not ask to die (Marker and Smith 1996, 84–85; Hendin, Rutenfrans, and Zylicz 1997; Keenan 1998, 17). The same is clear from the most recent report, which notes that in 2001 more than 25 percent of cases of euthanasia in The Netherlands were without request on the part of the person killed.[1]

None of this is compelling proof in itself against the legalization of PAS, but it is compelling proof that it is naïve to think that one can support the legalization of PAS and not, in effect, support the legalization of voluntary and of some kinds of nonvoluntary euthanasia. The same logic supports both.

The third reason PAS should not be legalized is the ever-present danger, especially in a time of necessary resource allocation, that PAS and active euthanasia would serve as a socially acceptable form of cost containment (Wolf 1996; Burt 1996, 169–72; New York State Task Force 1994, 143). The temptation to eliminate poverty by eliminating the poor might be hard to resist. It would be especially tempting to insurance companies, which might offer lower premiums to those who agree ahead of time to commit suicide if they are diagnosed with a terminal or chronic illness. Minority populations may perceive themselves to be especially vulnerable (King and Wolf 1998). And even if laws were passed forbidding such action, there would remain the inevitable subtle and not-so-subtle pressures exerted in families and even among the elderly themselves. the elderly see their peers agreeing to PAS or euthanasia in order eliminate a burden on their families, they may feel a responsibili do the same. Social and cultural pressures might become hard t st.

Because these same pressures already exist when it comes to refusing life-sustaining treatment, this argument is not itself totally compelling. That is the problem with "slippery slope" arguments. But there *is* a difference. PAS and euthanasia, once accomplished, are definitive, final choices. Decisions to forgo treatment can be changed if conditions warrant it. Perhaps of greater importance is the fact that people simply must have the legal right to be free from unwanted medical intervention; if we did not observe this right, we would needlessly increase suffering and attack personal autonomy. We do not want to go back to where we were. And so we grant this right, even though we know there can be cases in which unjust pressures are brought to bear on poor people to forgo treatment they may in fact want. We try to safeguard against this by insisting on criteria for surrogate decision making and by trying to be certain of what patients want. But the same is not true, I think, of PAS and euthanasia. The right to have help in killing oneself or the right to be killed is not an essential basic human right or human need. PAS would add further risks to those we already face in our current health care system, which discriminates against people unable to pay for their own care. It is a line we ought not cross.

Fourth, PAS should not be legal because the distinction between killing and allowing to die has been one of the pillars on which the present American consensus, which legally permits the forgoing of certain treatments, is based. The absolute legal prohibition of active euthanasia (and, thus far, the legal prohibition in most states of PAS) serves as a protective barrier against going too far and serves as a valid argument against those who think that forgoing treatment is itself euthanasia. If we remove that barrier, there may be fear on the part of some that we have gone too far already (Kamisar 1996, 495–96). There may, in other words, be a backlash against the present consensus that forgoing treatment is in many cases legally and morally right. The legalization of active euthanasia may lead politically to a restriction of the present consensus as the pendulum swings back.

There is already, in the court decisions we have examined, the kind of confusion that might lead to a strictly vitalistic legal code insisting on aggressive treatment for all people regardless of likely outcome. If the Second Circuit Court was right when it said that the equal protection clause required that we make no distinction between those on life support and those not on it, then perhaps, if we want to avoid euthanasia, we must insist on treating even against patients' wishes. If withholding or withdrawing treatment is itself euthanasia, as the Second Circuit implied, and as Justice Scalia explicitly claimed in *Cruzan*, then to avoid euthanasia we would have to refuse quite proper requests by patients or surrogates to withdraw life-sustaining treatment. Only by maintaining the distinction can we avoid this confusion.

And finally, PAS should remain illegal in order to preserve the integrity of the medical profession. Doctors are not now allowed to kill their patients. Permission to do this might possibly lead to mistrust. Admittedly, this can be said to beg the question. Those who support PAS argue that physicians would in this way be able to help their patients die and thus greater trust would result. But there is some evidence for concern here. In Australia, a law legalizing euthanasia in one section of the country was revoked, in part because Aboriginal peoples, fearing white doctors, worried that they would kill them. Similar fears are often found in minority populations in the United States (King and Wolf 1998).

Stage Four

My present judgment is not far removed from my judgment at stage three. Perhaps the difference is too minor to worry about, but the more aware I become of the possibilities of pain management, the more I think that, when proper pain control is available, it is morally wrong for people to request PAS or euthanasia. If I am right that legalizing physician-assisted suicide and euthanasia would be bad for our society, then, since even dying people have social responsibilities, dying people ought not further the move toward legalization by requesting this for themselves. I do not believe this moral obligation holds in some circumstances in which pain relief is not available. Thus in "deserted island" cases, and possibly in similar circumstances in developing nations (but I cannot know without knowing the likely social results of proposing a practice of euthanasia in those societies), euthanasia and assisted suicide may be morally right. It is true that in the United States pain relief is not always properly provided, but the answer in such cases is to insist on getting it, or to fire the doctor, or to change hospitals. There may be other exceptions in addition to the absence of pain relief, though I do not think they are many or common. So I continue to disagree with the judgment that active euthanasia and suicide are absolutely morally wrong. But the exceptions are rarer than I used to think they were, and I now, more than I once did, consider the dangers greater.

I am aware, as I have noted, that there is always a problematic remainder beyond pain, a remainder of "agent narrative suffering," loss of control, and family grief, which, at least arguably, only quick killing can eliminate. This remainder calls for care. It ought not be dismissed. But I do not think this remainder is enough to lead us to the judgment that active euthanasia and physician-assisted suicide are generally morally right. I am too worried about the social effects of the widespread practice of euthanasia. So even though it might be better for *me* to be killed now, or to kill myself now, rather than wait for death to come, it is better for *us* that I wait.

NOTE

1. This figure is from the "Van der Wal, Van der Maas Report," published on May 23, 2003. My source is an e-mail note to an online discussion group of moral theologians from Marie Vianney Bilgrien, "Re: Euthanasia in the Netherlands," May 23, 2003. The report states that in 2001 there were thirty-six hundred cases of euthanasia in The Netherlands, nine hundred of which were without request. See also Hendin (2003, 44), who claims, on the basis of the same figures, that "this is a system out of con-

trol." Theo A. Boer, a Dutch theologian, cites figures from earlier reports that also show a significant incidence of euthanasia performed without request (Boer 2003, 228). Bilgrien notes that this practice remains criminal manslaughter under the law in Holland, but Boer shows how easy it is for the requirements of the Dutch law to be ignored without serious consequence (Boer 2003, 236). There are other concerns as well, beyond the practice of euthanasia without request. For example, Dutch law allows for euthanasia to be requested by advance directive even before a terminal condition arises (Boer 2003, 227), which, given what we have seen about the problems connected with treatment directives, adds worry about proper interpretation. And there is evidence that hospitals and physicians are refusing to hire doctors who object to and will not practice euthanasia on their patients (Boer 2003, 234–35). Perhaps most worrisome about the practice of euthanasia in The Netherlands is the concern about extending its circumstances beyond terminal illness. The worry in Holland is not that the acceptance of physician-assisted suicide might lead to euthanasia, as is the concern in the United States, but that the acceptance of euthanasia might lead to the acceptance of assisted suicide. In Dutch usage, euthanasia implies a terminal illness, but assisted suicide does not. Some there now argue that since euthanasia is an accepted practice, there is no reason not to allow assistance at the suicide of persons who wish to end their lives because they are "finished with life" even though they are otherwise (physically) healthy (Boer 2003, 230–31). While the original law was supposed to be limited to cases of intractable suffering, palliative care in Holland has now significantly improved and supporters of euthanasia and assisted suicide now wish it extended to "psychological suffering, loneliness, fear of becoming socially redundant or irrelevant, fear of being a burden to relatives and loved ones, fear of insufficient care, fear of the time when no one calls you by your first name, Alzheimer's disease, as well as the fear of the prospect of Alzheimer's" (Boer 2003, 237). Boer notes the case of a psychiatrist who assisted at the suicide of a depressed woman without offering treatment for her depression; though found guilty, he was not punished because, apart from not ordering a psychiatric consult, he had behaved correctly (Boer 2003, 237). There is not yet any evidence of these practices in Oregon, but there is some concern that the privacy and secrecy controls imposed by the state health department are preventing the kinds of investigation that might disclose such problems (Moskowitz 2003).

—๛ *Chapter 8* ๛—

Medical Futility

W HEN I began working at St. Francis Medical Center in Pittsburgh in 1989, during a sabbatical year, I began with a number of preconceived notions about what I would find, some explicit and many implicit. One of these was that most instances of conflict about forgoing treatment between health care providers and patients or patient surrogates would be cases in which the providers would insist on initiating or continuing aggressive therapy while patients or, more often, patients' families would ask to have humanly useless or burdensome treatment withheld or withdrawn. The medical ethical literature I had read suggested that the paradigmatic case of conflict would set the physicians' medical model against the more humane moral sense of patients and families. Physicians, I anticipated, and possibly other health care providers, would see the main enemy as disease and death and thus try to hold it off at all costs. It would be the families who would ask that patients be allowed to die with dignity, free from disproportionate medication and technology.

What I found was more often the opposite. Though conflicts did and still do arise along the lines of this model, there had been a major shift in the type of conflictive case. The most contentious cases were usually those in which the families insisted on aggressive treatment while the physicians wanted to stop, often arguing that treatment was futile. From this context has arisen a debate about the meaning of and the criteria for "medical futility."

Professional discussions of medical futility began about 1988, but the word "futile" had been used before that, even though its exact meaning had not been specified. It is found in hospital policies on forgoing treatment. When used in these policies, *futile* refers generally to procedures that doctors are not required to offer because they are contrary to the standard of care; they are medically useless in a generally recognized way. Policies would simply note that physicians are never required to provide futile treatment. Only recently has there been argument as to what exactly that means. The medical futility debate has arisen because some have attempted to *expand* the notion of futility to include treatments that previously were not considered procedures doctors ought not provide. That is, treatments that physicians might have argued *for* in an era of physician paternalism, sometimes against the wishes of patients and families, are now to be rejected by physicians, against the wishes of patients and families, on the basis of futility. The question is whether or not this expansion is ethically justified. I argue that it is *not* justified.

The Importance of the Issue

In chapter 6, I discussed and argued against a movement that criticizes and would radically change the first pillar of the consensus concerning end-of-life treatment, the distinction between ordinary and extraordinary means of preserving life. It would do that by claiming that what has generally been seen as extraordinary and thus optional is really ordinary and thus mandatory. This challenge comes from the Right or the conservative political wing. In chapter 7, I discussed and argued against a movement that criticizes and would radically change the present American consensus by rejecting the legal and ethical notion that there is and ought to be a distinction between killing and allowing to die. Proponents of physician-assisted suicide and euthanasia would thus change (or eliminate) the second pillar of the present consensus. This challenge comes from the Left or the liberal political wing. The medical futility debate challenges the third pillar of the consensus, the procedural or legal pillar supporting the legal rights of patients or surrogates to decide about treatment options. It involves a proposal to allow physicians, on the basis of their medical knowledge, to reject certain treatments desired by patients or surrogates. Recent discussions have attempted to propose criteria for determining medical futility that would expand the applicability of this concept from its traditional restricted usage.

I have noted one indication of the importance of this topic: the shift from the older typical case in which the physician insists on aggressive treatment against the family's wishes to one in which the patient or family insists on treatment against the advice of the health care team. Why has this shift occurred? The number of articles dealing with the topic, especially in the 1980s and 1990s, indicates that it is a general phenomenon. Physicians and ethicists are increasingly interested in what to do when doctors want to stop and families want to treat. I believe, based on evidence from my own conversations with health care providers at various hospitals, that the shift first occurred in urban rather than rural hospitals. In rural hospitals physicians are still apt to insist on aggressive treatment for the terminally ill despite family wishes, whereas in urban hospitals conflicts tend to be the other way around. It is also possible that these changes began in the urban teaching centers and are now making their way to the rural institutions.

WHY THE SHIFT?

There are three causes for the growing concern about cases of this type and thus about medical futility. First, health care providers in the United States have become more aware of the importance of patient autonomy. There is a greater emphasis on informed consent and other issues of patients' rights. Certain decisions about treatment are made by the patient or the patient's surrogate, not by the physician or the health care team. One reason for this change was the general acceptance of a criticism made against the older, paternalistic approach. In 1973, Robert Veatch, one of the strongest critics of medical paternalism, attacked what he called the "generalization of expertise" (Veatch 1973), that is, the tendency of health care professionals, especially physicians, to assume that their considerable expertise in medicine gives them expertise as well in ethics and in determining correct values for their patients. Physicians are professionally trained to make medical decisions, he said (and I will argue that this includes decisions that a treatment is *medically futile*), but not necessarily to make decisions about what patients ought to do with respect to the values they cherish. The assumption that they can is a fallacy, the fallacy of generalization of expertise. Medical ethics has generally accepted this criticism of paternalism, as has recent U.S. law. Though it is true that patient autonomy cannot stand as an absolute value in automatic preference to all others—a point being made with increasing frequency, especially in the context of allocation of medical resources—the importance of autonomy is well recognized. Physicians have come to understand this. Legally and morally, the patient must be seen as more than a disease to be treated. The patient is also a person who makes decisions and whose values count.

It may seem puzzling to say that this is a reason for proposals that would reduce patient and surrogate authority by returning to health care professionals some of the decision-making authority that has been transferred since the 1960s to patients (and thus also to surrogates). But this change has brought with it a reduction in the automatic technological imperative that preceded it. Because physicians realize that patients and surrogates must enter into the decision-making process, they are more apt now than they used to be to hesitate before automatically going ahead with treatment. Perhaps ironically, therefore, the emphasis on patient autonomy has led to a situation in which physicians, no longer insisting on treatment in all cases, have begun in some cases to reject their patients' desires to continue aggressive treatment. There is also a growing sense that perhaps the American consensus has moved too far in the direction of the autonomy of the individual patient.

A second cause of the shift from cases in which providers insist on treating and patients or families refuse treatment to cases in which providers want to stop and families or patients insist on continuing is the ongoing increase in medical knowledge and the development of outcomes assessment. Health care providers are becoming more aware that certain procedures that initially showed great promise may not be appropriate in some specific clinical situations. This has quite properly contributed to a hesitation in performing procedures that physicians and nurses know will do little or no real good.

The third cause of the shift is more problematic: the developing restrictions on resources available to health care and to health care institutions. In the growing market-based approach to payment and insurance, hospitals often take serious losses by continuing treatment that family members wish but physicians consider unwarranted. Prospective payment schemes, such as diagnosis related groups (DRGs), in which hospitals are paid a set fee according to diagnosis, have largely replaced the retrospective fee-for-service approach in which doctors and institutions were paid for whatever they did. This has resulted in major hospital losses in cases in which families insist on treatment that physicians consider inappropriate. Physicians naturally defend the fiscal viability of the hospitals in which they work, and hospitals and health maintenance organizations (HMOs) put pressure on physicians to avoid needless treatments, because now the hospital, or the HMO, will take a loss if the cost of treatment exceeds repayment. Capitation schemes and other payment plans that penalize physicians who treat "too much" further bolster this disincentive to treat. Clearly this is a different financial incentive system from the one that formerly prevailed, which rewarded physicians for continuing aggressive treatment. Physicians find themselves more and more besieged by those who threaten their employment, usually implicitly but sometimes explicitly, if they spend "too much" on their patients. They are urged to decide against some treatments on the basis that they are unnecessary or futile.

The issue of medical futility is thus important because physicians are more and more arguing against treatment that patients or families want. And they are making the argument on the basis of medical futility.

THE *Wanglie* Case

A court case heard in Minnesota is typical of those involving the issue (*In re Wanglie*, 1991). It has been called "a case of Cruzan-in-reverse" ("Courting the Issues" 1991, 1). Hennepin County Medical Center went to court seeking to turn off Helga Wanglie's respirator and artificial nutrition. Like Nancy Cruzan, Helga Wanglie was in a persistent vegetative state. Her care was paid for by Medicare and an HMO, so the hospital was not losing money. Rather, it claimed that the treatment was medically inappropriate, though its legal claim was explicitly that Helga's husband, Oliver, ought not be the decision maker in the case. He insisted on continuing the treatment, arguing this on the basis of his and his wife's Lutheran beliefs, and what evidence there is suggests that Helga herself would have wanted the treatment continued. District court judge Patricia Belois decided in early July 1991 that Oliver Wanglie was the proper decision maker. The hospital did not appeal and continued life-sustaining treatment. Helga Wanglie died three days later, on July 4, 1991.

THE CONCEPT OF MEDICAL FUTILITY

With the *Wanglie* case as background, we turn to the issue of medical futility. What precisely is it, and what are the proper criteria for determining that a treatment is medically futile?

What the term means (or at least what it ought to mean) as a formal concept is quite simple. *Medical futility*, however its criteria are chosen, characterizes those treatments that must not be used because they are of no medical benefit to the patient. The treatment is, for this patient in this situation, contrary to the standard of medical care. Once a treatment has been categorized as medically futile, physicians must withhold it or withdraw it, regardless of the wishes of the patient or surrogate. This is a medical decision, not an ethical one, and it depends on the proper application of medical expertise. Physicians, not ethicists, patients, or patients' families, will apply the criteria of medical futility in individual cases.

The term is used, as I have stated, in policies on forgoing treatment and generally refers to treatments that doctors need not give. Policies might say simply that physicians need not provide "medically futile" or, simply, "futile" treatment. For example, the Forgoing Treatment Policy at the St. Francis Medical Center in Pittsburgh, written in 1990, reads: "If the requested treatment is clearly futile or non-beneficial, it need not be provided" (St. Francis Medical Center 1995, 6). What is almost certainly meant, though the lack of clarity makes it hard to prove this, is that futile treatment is treatment that provides no benefit at all.[1] The context of such policies supports the claim that futile treatment does not refer to life-sustaining treatment that does indeed maintain life but that some, or even most, people might not want. Those treatments, the policies would say, should be provided to patients who ask for them. Though not spelled out in any detail, whatever "futile" means, it means something that physicians are right to refuse.

Besides medically futile treatments, there are humanly futile treatments: morally extraordinary or optional treatments that some patients consider useless for themselves but others choose— for example, chemotherapy associated with a 25 percent chance of a two-year remission. But this kind of treatment was never considered futile in the sense that the treatment must never be given regardless of who wants it. Nor was, for example, hydration and nutrition for a permanently unconscious person considered futile in this sense, something that doctors must never do, something contrary to the standard of medical care.

In my judgment, then, when we use the term "medical futility," we ought to mean that a treatment thus characterized should never be offered regardless of who wants it. It is contrary to the standard of medical care. Doctors who offer or give it demonstrate that they are bad doctors. Only this formal definition of medical futility allows us to do anything with this concept that we cannot do with words we already have, such as "extraordinary" or "aggressive" or "unreasonable."

Doctors Do Have Expertise and Authority

I have already stated that I agree with Veatch's position criticizing the generalization of expertise. But this criticism does not mean that health care professionals have no expertise whatsoever. It does not mean that physicians are reduced to giving their patients a list of options and a bibliography of articles in the *New England Journal* and the *Annals of Internal Medicine*, telling them to go home, read up on it, and come back with a choice of treatment. Physicians, nurses, physicians' assistants, and other health care professionals are still the experts in medicine and health care, and unilateral decisions can be made, even without consulting the patient or the patient's surrogate.

A silly case makes this clear. If I go to a dialysis center with a head cold and demand dialysis as treatment, offer one thousand dollars in cash, insist that I am an autonomous person, quote from the literature against paternalism and the generalization of expertise, and threaten to sue if the center does not do what I want, the physician is required ethically and legally to refuse my request. I do not have any idea what I am talking about. Medical expertise must override my silly request. My demand contradicts the standard of care. There is no need to try to refer me to another physician or nurse who might (illegally and unethically) do what I ask. The dialysis center must simply tell me that dialysis is no treatment for my cold and send me away (unless there is reason to suspect I might be crazy and self-destructive, I suppose, and then one might try to get me committed for psychiatric observation).

Physicians have no obligation to give medically futile treatment to any patient. Indeed, they must *not* give it. They are not obliged to inform the patient or ask the patient's permission or that of the family. This applies to CPR, antibiotics, and all sorts of treatments that in other circumstances might be warranted.

Who Decides the Criteria for Medical Futility?

The criteria for determining medical futility are crucial. But are these criteria within the purview of medicine, ethics, or both? An analogy, though it is not perfect, will help here. A physician's expertise is needed to determine that a patient has died. In a case in which cardiopulmonary function is being maintained by machines after brain dysfunction has occurred, the expertise of a neurologist is needed. The neurologist runs tests to determine whether the criteria for total brain death have been met in any given case; if those criteria have been met, if total brain death has occurred, the patient is declared dead. The fact that relatives may say the patient has not yet died because they can see breathing is irrelevant. No further treatment is given. The decision is a medical one.

However, deciding what "kind" of brain death has occurred indicates that the determination of death was not and is not a purely medical one. As we noted in chapter 6, our society has decided that only total brain death means that a person is dead. We have rejected the arguments that irreversibly comatose people have already died. The cessation of all higher brain function is not enough, we have said, to allow us to declare a person dead. We do not want to bury breathing corpses—or to stop them from breathing and then bury them. This decision was an ethical and social one, not merely a medical one, though medical professionals had an important role to play in the discussion that led to the decision.

Now that the criteria are ethically and legally established, doctors are the ones who apply them. Doctors decide on the proper tests to use to determine if a person is or is not brain dead. But the establishment of what kind of brain dysfunction counts as death—that is, the establishment of the kinds of criteria used to determine that death has occurred—involves social, legal, and ethical decisions. This becomes clearer when we recall that there is still some discussion, largely in the context of organ procurement, concerning whether or not our nation ought to add anencephalics—those suffering from a congenital absence of most of the brain—and possibly the irreversibly comatose to the ranks of the truly dead. No one suggests that the American Academy of Neurology can, by itself, decree this kind of change.

The same applies to the issue of medical futility. Once a treatment is determined by the physician to be medically futile, the physician must not offer it or continue it. But the determination of the kinds of treatment that are going to be included in this category, that is, the determination of the kinds of criteria that must be met before medical futility is to be declared, is a societal, ethical, and legal issue, not a purely medical one.

Four Proposed Criteria

What are the criteria for determining when a treatment is medically futile? Stuart J. Youngner lists four criteria that might be proposed (Youngner 1988). I will argue that the first two are valid while the last two are not.

Physiological Uselessness

A treatment is clearly medically futile if it will fail in strictly physi-·ological terms. The dialysis will not clear the blood, the vasopressor will not increase the blood pressure, electric cardioversion will not start the heart, or arrhythmia control will not stop the fibrillation. Perhaps these procedures are tried and they fail. Perhaps, as in my silly dialysis example above, the treatment is entirely worthless considering the patient's condition. No one disagrees with this first criterion. In such circumstances, physicians must refuse to perform the procedure, regardless of patient or surrogate requests. Such a procedure is, in this case, contrary to the standard of medical care. It is medically futile.

Irrelevance to the Real Condition of a Dying Patient

A treatment is futile if, though it works in the direct or local physiological sense, it does not postpone death in a dying patient for even *a very short time*. The cardioversion does start the heart, but the heart stops again almost immediately and this happens each time CPR is done. The dialysis does clear the blood, but since the patient is immediately moribund from another cause, the dialysis is, in fact, irrelevant to the patient's underlying disease. A family member insists on knee surgery to remove a cartilage spur in a dying patient who will never leave the bed.

What counts as "a very short time"? If a ventilator will keep a dying patient alive for an extra day or two, but not longer, is use of it medically futile? If intubation or other intensive care unit (ICU) procedures will not reverse or even significantly affect the patient's "death spiral" but will probably postpone death for a day or two, can the physician refuse a request to admit to the ICU on the grounds that ICU treatment will not change the patient's "immediate dying" and is thus medically futile and violates the standard of medical care? There is no consensus about what constitutes immediate dying. I argue that dying in two or three days can *usually* be considered immediate dying, and hence the procedure in this case is usually medically futile. On the other hand, I would not consider death in two weeks or more immediate; in such a case, physicians could not unilaterally refuse a patient's or a surrogate's request for treatment. The intervening time of delay is less certain to me, and there is no clarity here in ethics or in law, though it seems most unlikely that any legal action would be successful against a physician who refused treatment when medical science clearly indicated that the treatment could not have prolonged the patient's life by as much as two weeks. But note that I have been careful here to add the word "usually" to my agreement that two or three days is "immediate dying." There may well be cases in which patients or families have valid reasons for asking that treatment attempt to extend life for that short time, as when family members are traveling to be with their loved one before death. So although I think it is clear that treatment that does not alter the patient's death spiral *at all,* that is, treatment that does *not* prolong life for even a very short time, is medically futile, I am not as sure about treatment that is likely to postpone dying for a day or two.

However, aside from the problem of what counts as a very short time, there is near universal agreement that if either of these criteria of futility are met, the futility is indeed "medical futility" and the physician must forgo the treatment. No consent by the patient is needed. The treatment is useless in the strictly medical sense, and the decision about its uselessness is made by the medical expert.

The third and fourth criteria are the ones around which the medical futility debate has centered. Those who propose an extension of the meaning of medical futility argue that they should be included. Those who, like me, oppose that extension, reject them.

Poor Quality of Life

A treatment is futile if it fails to meet the quality-of-life criterion. What if the treatment does indeed prolong physical life for a few weeks or longer but cannot lead to the patient's recovery? With treatment, the patient will not survive until discharge but is likely to survive for a time in the hospital. Or what if the treatment does result in discharge from the hospital but the patient's level of living is such that he or she cannot continue to carry out the basic purposes of life? What about the patient in a persistent vegetative state maintained for many years on medical nutrition and hydration?

Low Probability of Success

The treatment is futile if it has a low probability of success. What if the physician estimates that a treatment is 75 percent likely not to postpone dying, 20 percent likely to do so, though not until discharge, and only 5 percent likely to lead to discharge? In such cases, who makes the decision? Is this still the kind of futility that can properly be called medical futility, so that the physician may make a unilateral decision to forgo treatment?

DEBATE ABOUT THE CRITERIA

There has been considerable controversy in the literature about this question, though the amount of published research on the topic has decreased in the past few years.[2] One early article argued that a very low quality of life after a successful procedure or a very low probability of success should define treatment as medically futile (Schneiderman, Jecker, and Jonsen 1990). I reject this proposal.

I am convinced of the correct answer, an answer that generally has been accepted:[3] The health care professional, usually the attending physician, may decide unilaterally to withhold treatment when it is medically futile, and medical futility is based on the first two criteria I have noted, not on the last two. That is, treatment is medically futile if the answer to either of two questions is no. First, will the treatment do, in the immediate, specific, physiological sense, what it is intended to do? If the answer is no, it is medically futile and must not be given. Second, if the answer to the first question is yes, and if the patient's death is imminent, will the treatment and its resulting local, physiological effect cause a postponement of physical death? If the patient's death is imminent, and the treatment does not postpone physical death, even though it accomplishes in the local physiological sense what it is intended to accomplish (it purifies the blood, for example, or balances the electrolytes), the fact that physical death is not postponed by even a very short time means that the treatment is medically futile and should not be given. It is medically futile to treat a secondary and clinically unimportant symptom in a patient whose death is, from another cause, imminent.

There is, of course, an obvious exception to this. Treatment that relieves pain or other patient discomfort is not futile just because it does not postpone physical death. With this exception, however, these two questions can serve to define medical futility. Treatment that is futile for other reasons is not medically futile in this sense, and the decision to forgo it must be made only after consultation with the patient or surrogate, and only with his or her approval. Perhaps I want to be kept alive to see the Red Sox beat the Yankees—as they finally did in 2004—even though I know I will never leave the hospital. This reason may appeal only to someone from Massachusetts, but I am from that state and it does appeal to me. Or perhaps a patient wants to live until after the marriage of a son or daughter. This reason would, I think, appeal to most of us as a valid reason for resuscitation, even if the patient is virtually certain to die before leaving the hospital. Or perhaps a surrogate wants to continue treatment for religious reasons or even out of fear or guilt. Now the reason does not appeal to me. But the consensus in our nation is that this cannot be called medically futile treatment, and the decision to forgo treatment must not be made unilaterally by the physician, the health care team, or the hospital.

The other criteria that have been proposed, criteria three and four on Youngner's list, should be rejected as bases for medical futility, that is, as bases for the conclusion that physicians must unilaterally refuse to perform a procedure. As I have noted, some argue that in addition to the restrictive criteria I have supported, medical futility can be determined as well on the basis of the small probability of success and/or society's agreement that even a medically successful outcome is not humanly beneficial.[4] This set of criteria would enable physicians unilaterally to forgo treatment that had a minimal (perhaps less than 1 percent) chance of success and/ or, though medically successful, had an outcome most of us would not want for ourselves (for example, continuing life in a persistent vegetative state).

The "and/or" in the last paragraph is important. These two criteria could be conjunctive or disjunctive. That is, both could be required or either one could suffice. If both are required before a treatment can be said to be medically futile, then, although the definition of medical futility is thus expanded somewhat from the restrictive set of criteria I have suggested, it is not expanded as much as it would be if the proposed criteria were to be disjunctive. For example, if the criteria are conjunctive, nutrition and hydration for most patients in persistent vegetative states would not meet the criteria for medical futility. The treatment might be said to yield an outcome that most of us (the "reasonable person standard") would consider to be humanly undesirable. But the odds of reaching this medically successful outcome are great. With this conjunctive use of the proposed criteria, surrogates, not physicians, would still decide treatment. But if the criteria are disjunctive, if either would suffice as a basis for determining the medical futility of a proposed treatment, physicians could unilaterally choose to end nutrition for patients like Wanglie, Cruzan, or Schiavo, since a "reasonable person" would have decided that the outcome of their treatment was not truly beneficial. Under this disjunctive use, I might not get to see the Red Sox play, or a parent might not get to see a child married.

CONCLUSION ON THE CRITERIA

Criteria based on probability of success and societal determination of benefit ought not be used for declaring a treatment to be medically futile. Despite the literature that recommends this, physicians should not make unilateral decisions to forgo treatment on these bases. Patients and families should decide whether or not to forgo treatment with a small probability of success and/or with poor quality of life as a result of medical success. This means that though I do not agree with those who require hydration and nutrition for PVS patients, I do not think physicians should be empowered to reject such requests unilaterally. Such treatment may be morally extraordinary, humanly useless, or even silly or demeaning. But it is not *medically* futile.

Problems with this Restrictive Approach

The approach I propose to medical futility is very restrictive. Most treatments that providers rightly and humanely want to stop will not fit into my notion of medical futility. As the "Consensus Statement of the Society of Critical Care Medicine's Ethics Committee" puts it, "The concept of futility is generally not useful in establishing policies to limit treatment. Futile treatments, as we have defined them, are rare, and are usually not offered or disputed" (Ethics Committee 1997, 888). Some families will continue to demand aggressive therapy for very sick patients whom such procedures will keep alive but never truly benefit.

Physicians are often disturbed, even angered, by such requests. Why should patients and families think themselves capable of making these decisions? In the American context, part of the answer comes from the fact that for years many physicians and health care institutions supported a technological imperative: If treatment that could prolong a patient's life is available, that treatment ought to be tried, regardless of the quality of the outcome or the probability of success. In the American retrospective-payment (fee-for-service) context, in which the more a doctor or hospital did, the greater the profit, patients and families often found themselves unable to persuade health care providers to stop treatment. In all the early related court decisions in the United States, as I have noted, families asked that treatments be withdrawn and hospitals or physicians refused to do so.

But the ethical consensus and the law changed to allow patients and surrogates to make these choices. The Patient Self-Determination Act and advance directives, as well as state laws supporting them, added and still add to this shift in decision-making authority from doctors to patients. A social sense of which treatments ought to be implemented and which ought to be forgone has not emerged. Unlike many other nations, the United States has fostered an ethos of individual choice. Individuals, we believe, ought to be able to receive what they want. Although today's physicians and health care institutions are right to question patients' and surrogates' insistence that patients receive inappropriate treatments that are often costly and, at best, unlikely to be of benefit, it is important to recognize that the social context for this insistence is one that American medicine has supported and still supports. Other social contexts, such as those found in Europe in which a general society-wide vision of proper care prevails and in which access to health care is guaranteed and regulated by governments or other public bodies, provide to a better extent a basis for decision making at a higher, civic level. In these other contexts, individuals are less apt to feel they have a right to anything they request. Only systemic changes in American medicine will end the medical futility debate.

Reducing Demand for Inappropriate Treatment

The following are nine options that might reduce patient demand for inappropriate but not medically futile treatments (some of these would require the kind of systemic change America has thus far rejected):

1. Any system of national health insurance could rightly refuse to pay for such treatments. A good national health system will also specifically tell hospitals and providers that they need not give such treatments to patients who cannot pay for them. Unfortunately,

resistance to governmentally mandated single-payer universal coverage, exacerbated by televised political warnings of the horrors of government interference, makes such an alternative unlikely in the near future.

2. Private insurance companies, medical care organizations, preferred provider organizations, HMOs, and the like may also rightly refuse to pay for these treatments, though the legal implications of hospitals refusing to treat would be unclear without federal or state statutory indemnification. But because private insurers are ethically and legally required to tell their clients what treatments they will and will not pay for, and because health insurance in the United States is largely private and highly competitive, insurance companies are unlikely to refuse to cover inappropriate treatments. If one insurer told potential clients it would not pay for treatment that another covered, the former might be at a disadvantage in a market in which clients want access to all possible medical care.

3. Hospitals could establish public policies rejecting specific treatments in certain situations. A hospital might say, "We do not treat patients who are in a persistent vegetative state, because we believe the resources should go to our well-baby clinic instead." That is not a medical policy in the strict sense; rather, it is a social and ethical decision based on a wide range of factors including, but not limited to, the strictly medical. But hospitals are unlikely to take this approach, given possible damage to public relations in a competitive environment. Attempts by hospitals to establish "futility policies" are unlikely to define exactly which procedures will be unilaterally denied in which cases, and thus hospitals are likely to fall back on a policy that asks for better communication with patients (Wear et al. 1995) or a policy that admits of exceptions when, despite all attempts, families insist on continuing treatment (Saint John's Hospital 1995).

4. Hospitals or individual physicians can always go to court to find a guardian who will agree to forgo the inadvisable treatment. A judge is unlikely to rule in the hospital's or physician's favor,

however, unless it can be shown that either the surrogate is unfit because of a conflict of interest or the treatment is not only unreasonable but hurtful to the patient, which, with proper pain relief, should never be the case.[5]

5. Early review can often be helpful in reducing the number of cases of inappropriate treatment. If primary care physicians take the time to speak with their patients about these issues, many of these patients will opt against inappropriate treatment and perhaps leave advance directives that can help forestall such treatment later on. In this context, it is important to note that physicians act ethically when they advise patients and surrogates against procedures that offer little benefit. Health care providers are rightly expected by patients to give such advice. They are not supposed to behave as neutral observers who simply offer a list of options.

6. Time spent with the family can be of great help. It takes time for families to let go. Hospital personnel should try to keep families well informed of the deteriorating condition of patients. If the ICU attending physician tells a family on Monday that he hopes a series of diagnostic procedures will suggest a solution to an illness or injury, even though he knows that in this case a favorable prognosis is highly unlikely, and then the physician who comes in on Tuesday tells them that in this case there is no hope for recovery, it is hardly surprising that they are unable to let their loved one die. They want the Monday doctor back.

7. General education of the public is important. I am convinced that the medical community does significant harm with its competitive advertising. People are continually told only about the miracles that occur in hospitals. They naturally expect that another miracle is possible. And there is the problematic fact that medicine is not and can not be an exact science. The popular media is full of stories about patients whose cases were seemingly hopeless but who survived and even thrived. People naturally want that chance for themselves and their loved ones.

8. Living wills and durable powers of attorney may help families follow the expressed wishes of dying patients to forgo unreasonable

life-sustaining treatment. These documents, as we have seen, are most helpful in assuaging family guilt. Instead of having to decide *for* the patient, they can instead agree to do what the patient would want.

9. It is always correct for a physician or other provider to withdraw from a case if the treatment demanded is against his or her conscience, but the provision, as always, is that some other provider will agree to care for the patient, which is unlikely in this kind of situation.

Conclusion

In the light of recent legal decisions, and of the present American ethical consensus, physicians and other providers should not declare medical futility when a treatment would prolong the patient's life by any humanly significant length. Such treatment may well be inadvisable, too costly, silly, or even degrading. But this kind of quality-of-life decision should be made by the patient or the surrogate, not unilaterally by the physician. It is not strictly a medical decision, but a decision that includes ethical and social dimensions. Perhaps in the future, American support for individual decision making in health care will be balanced by a recognition of the needs of society and of the common good, but until systemic change occurs, the decision belongs to the patient.

Notes

1. But the coupling of the term "medically futile" with the less precise term "nonbeneficial" shows a lack of detailed development of the meaning. Indeed, the policy goes on to say that physicians who refuse to give such treatment, like those who object on ethical or religious grounds, may withdraw treatment but must transfer the patient to the care of another. The meaning that I am arguing for here would neither require nor permit such a transfer.

2. In addition to Youngner's work (1988), articles include Blackhall 1987 (which gives more latitude to physicians' unilateral decisions than I believe is appropriate); Tomlinson and Brody 1988 (make very helpful distinctions between medical futility and quality-of-life futility); Murphy 1988 (argues that physicians may unilaterally write a DNR order when the future quality of life is low [2100], a position I do not accept); Brennan 1988; Boyle 1988; Lantos et al. 1989; Paris, Crone, and Reardon 1990; Callahan 1991 (an approach similar to mine); Solomon 1993; Schneiderman, Faber-Langendoen, and Jecker 1994; Youngner 1994; Laffey 1996; Council on Ethical and Judicial Affairs 1999; Halevy 1999; and Helft, Siegler, and Lantos 2000.

3. This approach to medical futility is supported by the statement of the Ethics Committee of the Society of Critical Care Medicine (1997) and by the New York State Task Force on Life and the Law (1992, 195–204). It is also implied in the American Medical Association's statement (Council on Ethical and Judicial Affairs 1999). That published statement does not suggest that quality-of-life decisions may be made unilaterally by physicians. See also Helft, Siegler, and Lantos 2000. The authors note that the futility debate has largely ended because the attempt to expand the criteria has been medically, legally, and ethically unsuccessful. The authors also note that attempts at objectifying and quantifying outcomes of treatments have failed, thus making it difficult, if not impossible, to base decisions about quality of life and probability of success on clear and certain medical criteria. Attempts at designing medical futility policies have been process based and have rejected any unilateral decisions by physicians based on quality of outcome and probability of success, which of course is exactly what expanded medical futility is supposed to enable. The approach suggested here is also supported by Lantos et al. (1989), who argue that patients are best able to make decisions of this kind because their personal values and goals differ. Arthur Caplan rightly argues that the solution is not to use medical futility as a way to reject patient and family wishes but to increase the trust patients have in doctors (Caplan 1996). In her book-length treatment of the topic, Susan Rubin also argues against allowing unilateral decisions by physicians when patient values are at issue, but she seems also to reject even the most basic physiological understanding of medical futility, which in my judgment goes too far in rejecting physicians' competence to make medical decisions (Rubin 1998, 88–114).

4. These criteria are proposed in Schneiderman, Jecker, and Jonsen 1990. These authors argue that either a very small probability of medical success (less than 1 to 3 percent or no successes in the last one hundred cases) or an outcome that does not benefit the patient as a whole (the treatment only prolongs the life of an unconscious patient or the treatment maintains life but the patient remains dependent on intensive medical care) is sufficient for declaring a treatment medically futile. They wish these criteria to be independent, so that meeting either one is sufficient. They propose that nutritional support for a patient in a persistent vegetative state be considered medically futile and that physicians withhold or withdraw such support regardless of the wishes of the patient or the family (950). If medical care does not offer patients the opportunity to achieve any of life's goals, physicians must refuse to give it, regardless of the wishes of patients or surrogates (949, 952–53). In a later article written to answer critics, the authors admit that more empirical outcomes assessment is needed in order to support their proposed approach, but otherwise they continue to propose it (Schneiderman, Jecker, and Jonsen 1996).

5. The *Wanglie* case is one example. See also Helft, Siegler, and Lantos 2000, 295. These authors quote Daar 1995 as saying that almost every court case of this kind has been resolved in favor of the patient. They list one notable exception, *Gilgunn v. Massachusetts General Hospital* (1995), but that was a jury decision, not a court ruling. Alexander Morgan Capron analyzes this case and concludes that both judge and jury erred in applying the law; Mrs. Gilgunn's daughter's demand that treatment be maintained for her permanently comatose mother should have prevailed (Capron 1995).

GLOSSARY

advance directives. Declarations, usually written, made by competent people stating which treatments they would want (treatment directives or living wills) or which surrogates they would wish to make the decisions (proxy directives) if they themselves are later incapable of doing so.

allowing to die. The forgoing of life-sustaining treatment such that the patient is allowed to die of the underlying condition. It includes both withholding and withdrawing treatment. Contrast with killing. See also **pain control.**

autonomy. Self-rule. The principle or value of making decisions for oneself. One of the four basic principles.

beneficence. The principle or value of doing good, of benefitting others (including primarily though not solely the patient). One of the four basic principles.

best interests standard. Legally supported standard whereby decisions are made by a surrogate for an incompetent patient based on what is known or thought to be in the patient's interests (see also **substituted judgment standard**).

competency. Condition of a person whereby he or she is ethically or legally able to make decisions. Strictly, competency is determined by courts and thus the proper term is "decisional capacity," but "competency" is usually used. Most ethicists hold for a sliding scale of competency whereby persons who reject beneficial and nonburdensome life-sustaining treatments must be clearly competent to do so whereas minor decisions may be made by marginally competent persons. Determining competency is usually simple but can be very difficult.

confidentiality. The requirement that information gained in the therapeutic relationship not be given to those who have no right to it.

consultation. See **ethics consultation.**

cumulative legislation. A statutory law that is not intended to change or restrict existing rights or previous laws.

direct/indirect euthanasia (or **active/passive**). Older and confusing term whereby forgoing treatment is included as euthanasia and euthanasia includes not only killing but also allowing to die *Direct* or *active* means killing; *indirect* or *passive* means allowing to die, including certain cases of pain control. The distinction is often made according to the principle of double effect.

double effect principle. See **principle of double effect.**

durable power of attorney. Legal directive whereby a person appoints another to be attorney in fact with power to perform certain functions, including admission to hospitals, consent to treatment, and consent to forgo treatment, when that person becomes unable to do so. It is a form of proxy advance directive, sometimes used when states do not have an advance directive law that provides for appointment of a health care proxy.

ethics consultation. A consultation initiated by someone connected with a clinical case for getting advice concerning ethical issues, usually done by a team of members from the Institutional Ethics Committee.

euthanasia. Literally, in a wider sense, it means "good death" or "dying well." In its more usual, narrower sense, it is killing a terminally ill patient (see also **voluntary/nonvoluntary/involuntary** and **direct/indirect euthanasia**).

extraordinary means (of preserving life). Procedures whose burdens outweigh the benefits so that a patient has no moral obligation to accept them; morally optional treatment.

forgoing treatment. Withholding or withdrawing treatment.

informed consent. The process of giving necessary information to the patient or surrogate to enable that person to consent to or refuse to consent to treatment or the process of obtaining the consent.

informed consent form. The actual piece of paper that the patient signs. Not a legal substitute for informed consent.

justice. The principle or value of rendering to each person his or her due, of acting fairly, and including social distribution and allocation issues; one of the four basic principles.

killing. Actually doing something that kills or hastens death and is intended to do precisely that.

living will. See **advance directive.**

nonmaleficence. The principle or value of doing no harm, traditional in medical ethics; one of the four basic principles.

ordinary means (of preserving life). Procedures whose benefits outweigh the burdens to the extent that a patient has a moral obligation to accept them; morally obligatory treatment.

pain control. Relief of pain, usually by pharmacological agent. Ethically and legally pain may and, if the proper decision maker agrees, must be eliminated in a dying patient, even if this contributes causally to the hastening of death, provided no one intends (wants as an end to be chosen for its own sake) that the patient die and provided the amount and means of delivery of the agent are such that they are proper for the elimination of pain.

palliative support. Treatment aimed at relieving pain and suffering rather than sustaining the patient's life.

palliative support care orders form. The form used by physicians to order palliative support and to order the forgoing of certain life-sustaining treatments, based on the informed consent of patient or surrogate.

paternalism (or **parentalism**). Choosing (treatment) for others on the basis of their good whether or not they want it; opposed to autonomy.

Patient Self-Determination Act (PSDA). The federal law requiring that admitted patients be informed about hospital policy and state law concerning forgoing treatment, that they be asked about their advance directives, and that these be recorded if they are available.

persistent vegetative state (PVS). A condition usually caused by oxygen deprivation to the cerebral cortex (higher brain) resulting in total and irreversible inability to perform internal or external conscious acts. PVS patients undergo sleep-wake cycles (eyes open and close) and other movements directed by the brain stem but are unaware of these movements or of themselves or anything around them.

physician-assisted suicide. Patient-chosen and patient-accomplished suicide with the direct and formal help of the physician, usually by prescribing drugs and informing the patient how much to take to accomplish the suicide. Illegal in most states. The Oregon law permitting it was implicitly found constitutional by the Supreme Court;

circuit court decisions concluding that laws forbidding it are unconstitutional were later reversed by the Court.

principle of double effect. A principle with four conditions claiming to determine when actions with both good and bad effects are morally right or wrong.

proxy directive. See **advance directive.**

substituted judgment standard. A legally supported standard whereby decisions are made by a surrogate for a now-incompetent patient based on what the patient is known to have wanted (see also **best interests standard**).

surrogate. A proper decision maker for an incompetent patient. Usually members of the family, sometimes a proxy appointed by advance directive, least often a court-appointed guardian.

terminal illness (or **condition**). In a stricter sense, usually incorporated into advance directive laws, this is a condition from which a person will, in the reasonable judgment of physicians, almost certainly die in a short time, even if aggressive medical interventions are done. In this sense PVS, for example, is not a terminal condition, since nutrition can prolong physical life. In the larger sense usually preferred by philosophers and theologians, this is a condition from which a person will almost certainly die, prescinding from the question of medical intervention. In this sense PVS is a terminal condition. The difference is often important in distinguishing between killing and allowing to die and in interpreting advance directive laws.

voluntary/nonvoluntary/involuntary euthanasia. Distinguished according to whether the patient actually asks to be killed/cannot ask but is killed by surrogate decision/asks not to be killed but is killed anyway. See **euthanasia.**

withholding treatment. Deciding to not begin treatment.

withdrawing treatment. Deciding to stop treatment that has been begun. Ethically and legally, if all other factors are equal, it is the same as withholding.

CASES CITED

Brophy v. New Eng. Sinai Hospital, Inc., 497 N.E.2d 626 (Mass. 1986)

Bush v. Schiavo, 885 So.2d 321 (Fla. 2004)

Compassion in Dying v. Washington, 79 F.3d 790 (9th Cir. 1996)

Cruzan v. Director, 497 U.S. 261 (1900)

Doe v. Bolton, 410 U.S. 179 (1973)

Gilgunn v. Massachusetts General Hospital, No. SUC 92-4820 (Super. Ct. Suffolk County, Mass., 22 April 1995)

Griswold v. Connecticut, 381 U.S. 479 (1965)

In re Conroy, 98 N.J. 321, 486 A.2d 1209 (N.J. 1985)

In re Doe, 45 Pa. D. & C. 3d 371 (C.P. Phila. County 1979)

In re Eichner, 423 N.Y.S.2d 580 (Sup. Ct. Nassau County 1979)

In re Fiori, 673 A.2d 905 (Pa. 1996)

In re Guardianship of Schiavo, 851 So.2d 182 (Fla. 2d Dist. Ct. App. 2003)

In re Jobes, 529 A.2d 434 (N.J. 1987)

In re Quinlan, 335 A.2d 647 (N.J. 1976)

In re Wanglie, No. PX-91-283 (Minn. 4th Dist. Ct. Hennepin County, 1 July 1991)

Martin v. Martin, 538 N.W.2d 399 (Mich. 1995)

McConnell v. Beverly Enters.-Conn., Inc., 533 A.2d 596 (Conn. 1989)

Planned Parenthood v. Casey, 505 U.S. 833 (1992)

Quill v. Vacco, 80 F.3d 716 (2d Cir. 1996)

Roe v. Wade, 410 U.S. 113 (1973)

Schiavo ex rel. Schindler v. Schiavo, No. 8:05-CV-530-T-27TBM (M.D. Fla. Mar. 22, 2005)

Superintendent of Belchertown State Sch. v. Saikewicz, 370 N.E.2d 417 (Mass. 1977)

Vacco v. Quill, 117 S.Ct. 2293 (1997)

Washington v. Glucksberg, 117 S.Ct. 2258 (1997)

Webster v. Reproductive Health Services, 492 U.S. 490 (1989)

Wendland v. Wendland, 110 Cal.Rptr.2d 412 (2001)

REFERENCES

American Academy of Neurology. 1989. "Position of the American Academy of Neurology on Certain Aspects of the Care and Management of the Persistent Vegetative State Patient." *Neurology* 39 (January): 125–26.

American College of Physicians. 1990. "Life, Death, and the American College of Physicians: The Cruzan Case." *Annals of Internal Medicine* 112:802–4.

American Medical Association. 1986. *Current Opinions.* Chicago: American Medical Association.

Annas, George J. 1986. "Do Feeding Tubes Have More Rights than Patients?" *Hastings Center Report* 16, no. 1 (February): 26–28.

———. 1996. "The Promised End: Constitutional Aspects of Physician-Assisted Suicide." *Legal Issues in Medicine* 335, no. 9 (August 29): 683–87.

———. 2005. "Culture of Life: Politics at the Bedside—the Case of Terri Schiavo." *New England Journal of Medicine* 352, no. 16 (April 21): 1710–15.

Ashley, Benedict, and Kevin D. O'Rourke. 1997. *Health Care Ethics: A Theological Analysis.* 4th ed. Washington, DC: Georgetown University Press.

Baron, Charles H. 2006. "Not DEA'd Yet: *Gonzales v. Oregon.*" *Hastings Center Report* 36, no. 2 (March–April): 8.

Beauchamp, Tom L., and James F. Childress. 2001. *Principles of Biomedical Ethics.* 5th ed. Oxford: Oxford University Press.

Billings, J. Andrew. 1985. "Comfort Measures for the Terminally Ill: Is Dehydration Painful?" *Journal of the American Geriatrics Society* 33 (11): 808–10.

Blackhall, Leslie J. 1987. "Must We Always Use CPR?" *New England Journal of Medicine* 317, no. 20 (November 12): 1281–85.

Boer, Theo A. 2003. "After the Slippery Slope: Dutch Experiences on Regulating Active Euthanasia." *Journal of the Society of Christian Ethics* 23, no. 2 (Fall/Winter): 225–42.

Bone, Roger C., E. C. Rackow, J. G. Weg, and members of the ACCP/SCCM Consensus Panel. 1990. "Ethical and Moral Guidelines for the Initiation, Continuation, and Withdrawal of Intensive Care." *Chest* 97:952–53, 955.

Boyle, Philip J. 1988. "DNR and the Elderly." *Issues in Health Care, St. Louis Univ. Medical Center for Health Care Ethics*, December.

Brennan, Troyen A. 1988. "Incompetent Patients with Limited Care in the Absence of Family Consent." *Annals of Internal Medicine* 109 (November 15): 819–25.

Bresnahan, James F., and James F. Drane. 1986. "A Challenge to Examine the Meaning of Living and Dying." *Health Progress* 67, no. 10 (December): 32–37, 98.

Burke, Greg. 2001a. "Reply to 'A Necessary Tension.'" *Ethics & Medics* 26, no. 8 (August): 2–3.

————. 2001b. "Tube Feeding and Advanced Dementia." *Ethics & Medics* 26, no. 3 (March): 1–2.

Burke, Raymond L. 2005. "The Evil of So-Called Euthanasia." Bishop's statement.

Burt, Robert A. 1996. "Constitutionalizing Physician-Assisted Suicide: Will Lightening Strike Thrice?" *Duquesne Law Review* 35, no. 1 (Fall): 159–81.

Cahill, Lisa Sowle. 2006. "Notes on Moral Theology: Bioethics." *Theological Studies* 67, no. 1 (March): 120–42.

Callahan, Daniel. 1991. "Medical Futility, Medical Necessity: The-Problem-Without-a-Name." *Hastings Center Report* 21, no. 4 (July–August): 30–35.

Caplan, Arthur L. 1996. "Odds and Ends: Trust and the Debate over Medical Futility." *Annals of Internal Medicine* 125 (October 15): 688–89.

Capron, Alexander Morgan. 1995. "Abandoning a Waning Life." *Hastings Center Report* 25, no. 4 (July–August): 24–26.

Carson, Ronald A. 1989. "The Symbolic Significance of Giving to Eat and Drink." In *By No Extraordinary Means: The Choice to Forgo Life-Sustaining Food and Water*, edited by Joanne Kynn. Bloomington: Indiana University Press.

Catechism of the Catholic Church. 1994. Mahwah, NJ: Paulist Press.

Catholic Health Association. 2004. Statement on the March 20, 2004, Papal Allocution. www.chausa.org.

Catholic Health Association of Wisconsin. 1989. *Nutrition and Hydration Guidelines*. Madison: Catholic Health Association of Wisconsin, March.

Chiong, Winston. 2005. "Brian Death without Definitions." *Hastings Center Report* 35, no. 6 (November–December): 20–30.

Congregation for the Doctrine of the Faith, 1980. 1998. "Declaration on Euthanasia." In *On Moral Medicine: Theological Perspectives in Medical Ethics*, edited by Stephen E. Lammers and Allen D. Verhey, 650–55. 2nd ed. Grand Rapids, MI.: William B. Eerdmans.

Council on Ethical and Judicial Affairs of the American Medical Association. 1999. "Medical Futility in End-of-Life Care." *Journal of the American Medical Association* 281:937–41.

"Courting the Issues: Decisions in Minnesota and Missouri." 1991. *Hospital Ethics* 7, no. 2 (March–April): 1–5.

Cronin, Daniel A. 1958. *The Moral Law in Regard to the Ordinary and Extraordinary Means of Conserving Life*. Rome: Pontifical Gregorian University.

Daar, J. F. 1995. "Medical Futility and Implications for Physician Autonomy." *American Journal of Law and Medicine* 21:221–40.

deBlois, Jean, and Kevin D. O'Rourke. 1995. "Issues at the End of Life: The Revised *Ethical and Religious Directives* Discuss Suicide, Euthanasia, and End-of-Life Procedures." *Health Progress* 76, no. 8 (November–December): 24–27.

Derr, Patrick G. 1986. "Why Food and Fluids Can Never Be Denied." *Hastings Center Report* 16, no. 1 (February): 28–30.

Devine, Richard J. 1989. "Save the Body, Lose the Soul." *Health Progress*, June, 68–72.

Diamond, Eugene F. 2002. "Resuscitation and the Operating Room." *Ethics & Medics* 27, no. 5 (May): 3–4.

Doerflinger, Richard M. 1999. "An Uncertain Future for Assisted Suicide." *Hastings Center Report* 29, no. 1 (January–February): 52.

Dombi, William A. 2005. Lessons from Schiavo beyond the Legal. *Caring* 24, no. 5 (May): 28–30.

Dorff, Elliot N. 2000. "End-Stage Medical Care: Practical Applications." In *Life and Death Responsibilities in Jewish Biomedical Ethics*, edited by Aaron L. Mackler, 338–58. New York: Jewish Theological Seminary of America.

Dresser, Rebecca. 2002. "The Conscious Incompetent Patient." *Hastings Center Report* 32, no. 3 (May–June): 9–10.

———. 2005. "Schiavo's Legacy: The Need for an Objective Standard." *Hastings Center Report* 35, no. 3 (May–June): 20–22.

Eberl, Jason T. 2005. "Extraordinary Care and the Spiritual Goal of Life: A Defense of the View of Kevin O'Rourke, O.P." *National Catholic Bioethics Quarterly* 5, no. 3 (Autumn): 491–501.

Ethics Committee of the Society of Critical Care Medicine. 1997. "Consensus Statement of the Society of Critical Care Medicine's Ethics Committee Regarding Futile and Other Possibly Inadvisable Treatments." *Critical Care Medicine* 25 (5): 887–91.

Fagerlin, Angela, and Carl E. Schneider. 2004. "Enough: The Failure of the Living Will." *Hastings Center Report* 34, no. 2 (March–April): 30–42.

Feldman, David F. 1986. *Health and Medicine in the Jewish Tradition*. New York: Crossroad.

Fins, Joseph J. 2005. "Rethinking Disorders of Consciousness: New Research and Its Implications." *Hastings Center Report* 35, no. 2 (March–April): 22–24.

Finucane, Thomas E., Colleen Christmas, and Kathy Travis. 1999. "Tube Feeding in Patients with Advanced Dementia: A Review of the Evidence." *Journal of the American Medical Association* 282, no. 14 (October 13): 1365–70.

Florida Catholic Conference. 2005. "Florida Bishops Urge Safer Course for Terri Schiavo." www.flacathconf.org/Publications/BishopsStatements/Bpst2000/TerriSchiavo.htm.

Flynn, Eileen P. 1990. *Hard Decisions: Forgoing and Withdrawing Artificial Nutrition and Hydration.* Kansas City, MO: Sheed & Ward.

Ford, Norman M. 2005. "Thoughts on the Papal Address and MANH." *Ethics & Medics* 30, no. 2 (February): 3–4.

Furton, Edward J. 2005. "Nutrition and Hydration: To the Editor." *Hastings Center Report* 35, no. 3 (May–June): 5.

Gert, Heather J. 2002. "Avoiding Surprises: A Model for Informing Patients." *Hastings Center Report* 32, no. 4 (September–October): 23–32.

Gillick, Muriel R. 2000. "Rethinking the Role of Tube Feeding in Patients with Advanced Dementia." *New England Journal of Medicine* 342, no. 3 (January 20): 206–10.

Grisso, Thomas, and Paul S. Applebaum. 1998. *Assessing Competence to Consent to Treatment.* New York: Oxford University Press.

Halevy, Amir. 1999. "Medical Futility in End-of-Life Care." *Journal of the American Medical Association* 282, no. 14 (October 13): 1331–32.

Hartman, Rhonda Gay. 2000. "Adolescent Autonomy: Clarifying an Ageless Conundrum." *Hastings Law Journal* 51, no. 6 (August): 1265–1362.

———. 2001. "Adolescent Decisional Autonomy for Medical Care: Physician Perceptions and Practices." *University of Chicago Law School Roundtable* 8 (1): 87–134.

Hastings Center. 1987. *Guidelines on the Termination of Life-Sustaining Treatments and the Care of the Dying.* Briarcliff Manor, NY: Hastings Center.

Helft, Paul R., Mark Siegler, and John Lantos. 2000. "The Rise and Fall of the Futility Movement." *New England Journal of Medicine* 343, no. 4 (July 27): 293–95.

Hendin, Herbert. 2003. "The Practice of Euthanasia." *Hastings Center Report* 33, no. 4 (July–August): 44–45.

Hendin, Herbert, Chris Rutenfrans, and Zbigniew Zylicz. 1997. "Physician-Assisted Suicide and Euthanasia in the Netherlands." *Journal of the American Medical Association* 277, no. 21 (June 4): 1720–22.

Hyun, Insoo. 2002. "Waiver of Informed Consent, Cultural Sensitivity, and the Problem of Unjust Families and Traditions." *Hastings Center Report* 32, no. 5 (September–October): 14–22.

"In Re Quinlan." 1982. In *Law and Bioethics: Texts with Commentary on Major U.S. Court Decisions.* 1982. Edited by Thomas A. Shannon and Jo Ann Manfra, 147–72. New York: Paulist Press.

Janssens, Louis. 1983. "Transplantations d'Organes." *Foi et Temps* 4:308–24.

John Paul II. 2004. "Care for Patients in a 'Permanent Vegetative State.'" *Origins* 33, no. 43 (April 8): 738–40.

Kahlenborn, Chris. 2001. "A Necessary Tension and Tube Feeding." *Ethics & Medics* 26, no. 8 (August): 1–2.

Kamisar, Yale. 1996. "'The 'Right to Die': On Drawing (and Erasing) Lines." *Duquesne Law Review* 35, no. 1 (Fall): 481–521.

Keenan, James F. 1998. "The Case for Physician-Assisted Suicide?" *America,* November 14, 14–19.

Kelly, David F. 1979. *The Emergence of Roman Catholic Medical Ethics in North America: An Historical—Methodological—Bibliographical Study.* New York: Edwin Mellen Press.

———. 1988. "Individualism and Corporatism in a Personalist Ethics: An Analysis of Organ Transplants." In *Personalist Morals,* edited by J. Selling, 147–65. Leuven, Belgium: Leuven University Press.

———. 1991. *Critical Care Ethics: Treatment Decisions in American Hospitals.* Kansas City, MO: Sheed & Ward.

———. 2004. *Contemporary Catholic Health Care Ethics.* Washington, DC: Georgetown University Press.

Kelly, Gerald. 1950. "The Duty of Using Artificial Means of Preserving Life." *Theological Studies* 11:203–20.

———. 1958. *Medico-Moral Problems.* St. Louis: Catholic Hospital Association of the United States and Canada.

King, Patricia A., and Leslie E. Wolf. 1998. "Lessons for Physician-Assisted Suicide from the African-American Experience." In *Physician-Assisted Suicide: Expanding the Debate*, edited by Margaret D. Batten, Rosamond Rhodes, and Anita Silvers, 91–112. New York: Routledge.

Laffey, Judy. 1996. "Bioethical Principles and Care-Based Ethics in Medical Futility." *Cancer Practice* 4, no. 1 (January–February): 41–46.

Lantos, John D., Peter A. Singer, Robert M. Walker, Gregory P. Gramelspacher. 1989. "The Illusion of Futility in Clinical Practice." *American Journal of Medicine* 87:81–84.

"The Latest Word: Brophy Dies." 1986. *Hastings Center Report* 16, no. 6 (December): 32.

"The Latest Word: In the Courts." 1986. *Hastings Center Report* 16, no. 5 (October): 47.

Latkovic, Mark S. 2005. "The Morality of Tube Feeding PVS Patients: Critique of the View of Kevin O'Rourke, O.P." *National Catholic Bioethics Quarterly* 5, no. 3 (Autumn): 503–13.

Liebrecht, John. 1990. "The Nancy Cruzan Case." *Origins* 19, no. 32 (January 11): 525–26.

Mackler, Aaron L. 2003. *Introduction to Jewish and Catholic Bioethics: A Comparative Analysis*. Washington, DC: Georgetown University Press.

Maguire, Daniel C. 1974. *Death by Choice*. Garden City, NY: Doubleday.

Mappes, Thomas A. 2003. "Persistent Vegetative State, Prospective Thinking, and Advance Directives." *Kennedy Institute of Ethics Journal* 13, no. 2 (June): 119–39.

Marker, Rita L., and Wesley J. Smith. 1996. "The Art of Verbal Engineering." *Duquesne Law Review* 35, no. 1 (Fall): 81–107.

May, William E. 1998. "Tube Feeding and the Vegetative State." *Ethics & Medics* 23, no. 12 (December): 1–2.

———. 1999. "Tube Feeding and the Vegetative State." *Ethics & Medics* 24, no. 1 (January): 3–4.

May, William E., Robert Barry, Orville Griese, Germain Grisez. 1987. "Feeding and Hydrating the Permanently Unconscious and Other Vulnerable Persons." *Issues in Law and Medicine* 3 (3): 204–11.

May, William F. 1983. *The Physician's Covenant: Images of the Healer in Medical Ethics*. Philadelphia: Westminster Press.

McCartney, James J. 1986. "Catholic Positions on Withholding Sustenance for the Terminally Ill." *Health Progress,* October, 38–40.

McCormick, Richard A.1992. "'Moral Considerations' Ill Considered." *America* 166, no. 9 (March 14): 210–14.

McCormick, Richard A., and John J. Paris. 1987. "The Catholic Tradition on the Use of Nutrition and Fluids." *America* 156:358.

McFadden, Charles J. 1961. *Medical Ethics.* 5th ed. Philadelphia: F. A. Davis.

McHugh, James. 1989. "Artificially Assisted Nutrition and Hydration." *Origins* 19, no. 19 (October 12): 314–16.

Meisel, Alan. 1989. *The Right to Die.* New York: John Wiley & Sons.

———. 1995. *The Right to Die.* 2nd ed. 2 vols. New York: John Wiley & Sons.

———. 2003. *The Right to Die, 2nd Edition 2003 Supplement.* New York: Aspen Publishers.

Miles, Steven H., and Allison August. 1990. "Courts, Gender and the Right to Die." *Law, Medicine and Health Care* 18, nos. 1–2 (Spring–Summer): 85–95.

Miller, Franklin G., and Diane E. Meier. 1998. "Voluntary Death: A Comparison of Terminal Dehydration and Physician-Assisted Suicide." *Annals of Internal Medicine* 128, no. 7 (April 1): 559–62.

Morlino, Robert C. 2005. "Medical Treatment: Make Decisions Based on Catholic Teaching." Bishop's statement.

Moskowitz, Ellen. 2003. "The Consensus on Assisted Suicide." *Hastings Center Report* 33, no. 4 (July–August): 46–47.

Mulligan, James J. 2005. "Caring for the Unconscious." *Ethics & Medics* 30, no. 7 (July): 2–4.

Multi-Society Task Force on PVS. 1994. "Medical Aspects of the Persistent Vegetative State." *New England Journal of Medicine* 330, nos. 21 and 22 (May 26 and June 2): 1499–1508, 1572–79.

Munsat, Theodore L., William H. Stuart, and Ronald E. Cranford. 1989. "Guidelines on the Vegetative State: Commentary on the American Academy of Neurology Statement." *Neurology* 39:123–24.

Murphy, Donald J. 1988. "Do-not-Resuscitate Orders: Time for Reappraisal in Long-Term-Care Institutions." *Journal of the American Medical Association* 260, no. 14 (October 14): 2098–2101.

National Conference of Catholic Bishops. 1995. *Ethical and Religious Directives for Catholic Health Care Services.* Washington, DC: United States Catholic Conference.

Neher, Jon O. 2004. "Like a River." *Hastings Center Report* 34, no. 2 (March–April): 9–10.

Nelson, Lawrence J. 2003. "Persistent Indeterminate State: Reflections on the Wendland Case." *Issues in Ethics* 14, no. 1 (Winter): 14–17.

New York State Task Force on Life and the Law. 1992. *When Others Must Choose: Deciding for Patients Without Capacity.* New York: New York State Task Force on Life and the Law.

———. 1993. *When Others Must Choose: Deciding for Patients Without Capacity: Supplement to Report and Legislation.* New York: New York State Task Force on Life and the Law.

———. 1994. *When Death Is Sought: Assisted Suicide and Euthanasia in the Medical Context.* New York: New York State Task Force on Life and the Law.

Oregon and Washington Bishops. 1991. "Living and Dying Well." *Origins* 21, no. 22 (November 7): 346–52.

Oregon Death with Dignity Act. 1998. In *Physician-Assisted Suicide: Expanding the Debate*, edited by Margaret D. Batten, Rosamond Rhodes, and Anita Silvers, 443–48. New York: Routledge, 1998.

O'Rourke, Kevin D. 1989. "Father Kevin O'Rourke on Hydration and Nutrition: Open Letter to Bishop McHugh." *Origins* 19, no. 21 (October 26): 351–52.

———. 1999. "On the Care of 'Vegetative' Patients: A Response to William E. May's 'Tube Feeding and the "Vegetative State."'" *Ethics & Medics* 24, nos. 4 and 5 (April and May): 3–4, 3–4.

———. 2005. "The Catholic Tradition on Forgoing Life Support." *National Catholic Bioethics Quarterly* 5, no. 3 (Autumn): 537–53.

O'Rourke, Kevin D., and Jean deBlois. 1992. "Removing Life Support: Motivations, Obligations: An Opinion on NCCB Committee for Pro-

Life Activities' Statement on Artificial Hydration and Nutrition." *Health Progress*, July–August, 20–27, 38.

Paris, John J. 1986. "When Burdens of Feeding Outweigh Benefits." *Hastings Center Report* 16, no. 1 (February–March): 30–32.

Paris, John J., Robert K. Crone, and Frank Reardon. 1990. "Physicians' Refusal of Requested Treatment: The Case of Baby L." *New England Journal of Medicine* 322, no. 14 (April 5): 1012–15.

Pennsylvania Bishops. 1992. "Nutrition and Hydration: Moral Considerations." *Origins* 21, no. 34 (January 30): 541, 543–53.

Pius XII. 1958. "The Prolongation of Life: An Address of Pope Pius XII to an International Congress of Anesthesiologists" (1957). Reprinted in *The Pope Speaks* 4, no. 4 (Spring): 393–98.

Pollock, David S., and Todd M. Begg. 1990. "The Constitutional Right to Die." Pittsburgh: Pollock and Adams.

President's Commission for the Study of Ethical Problems in Medicine and Biomedical and Behavioral Research. 1983. *Deciding to Forego Life-Sustaining Treatment*. Washington, DC: GPO.

Printz, Louise A. 1989. "Withholding Hydration in the Terminally Ill: Is It Valid?" *Geriatric Medicine*, April, 81–84.

Quill, Timothy E. 2005. "Terri Schiavo: A Tragedy Compounded." *New England Journal of Medicine* 352, no. 16 (April 21): 1630–31, 1633.

Repenshek, Mark, and John Paul Slosar. 2004. "Medically Assisted Nutrition and Hydration: A Contribution to the Dialogue." *Hastings Center Report* 34, no. 6 (November–December): 13–16.

Rothenberg, Leslie Steven. 1986. "The Dissenting Opinions: Biting the Hands that Won't Feed." *Health Progress*, December, 38–45, 99.

Rubin, Susan B. 1998. *When Doctors Say No: The Battleground of Medical Futility*. Bloomington: Indiana University Press.

Saint John's Hospital and Health Center. 1995. *Policy: Ethically Appropriate and Inappropriate Medical Treatment, and Related Matters*. Santa Monica, CA: St. John's Hospital and Health Center.

Schneider, Carl E. 1997. "Making Sausage: The Ninth Circuit's Decision." *Hastings Center Report* 27, no. 1 (January–February): 27–28.

———. 2004. "Benumbed." *Hastings Center Report* 34, no. 1 (January–February): 9–10.

Schneiderman, Lawrence J., Kathy Faber-Langendoen, and Nancy S. Jecker. 1994. "Beyond Futility to an Ethic of Care." *American Journal of Medicine* 92:110.

Schneiderman, Lawrence J., Nancy S. Jecker, and Albert R. Jonsen. 1990. "Medical Futility: Its Meaning and Ethical Implications." *Annals of Internal Medicine* 112, no. 12 (June 15): 949–54.

———. 1996. "Medical Futility: Response to Critiques." *Annals of Internal Medicine* 125 (October 15): 669–74.

Shannon, Thomas A., and James J. Walter. 1988. "The PVS Patient and the Forgoing/Withdrawing of Medical Nutrition and Hydration." *Theological Studies* 49, no. 4 (December): 623–47.

———. 2004. "Implications of the Papal Allocution on Feeding Tubes." *Hastings Center Report* 34, no. 4 (July–August): 18–20.

———. 2005a. "Assisted Nutrition and Hydration and the Catholic Tradition." *Theological Studies* 66, no. 3 (September): 651–62.

———. 2005b. "Nutrition and Hydration: Shannon and Walter Reply." *Hastings Center Report* 35, no. 3 (May–June): 5.

———. 2005c. "Nutrition and Hydration: To the Editor." *Hastings Center Report* 35, no. 3 (May–June): 4.

Soloman, Mildred Z. 1993. "How Physicians Talk About Futility: Making Words Mean Too Many Things." *Journal of Law, Medicine & Ethics* 21:231–37.

SSM Health Care System. 1989. "Continuing or Discontinuing Treatment: Ethical Criteria: Catholic Health-Care System's Brief." *Origins* 19, no. 17 (September 28): 279–86.

St. Francis Medical Center. 1995. *Forgoing Treatment Policy.* Pittsburgh: St. Francis Medical Center.

Texas Bishops. 1990. "On Withdrawing Artificial Nutrition and Hydration." *Origins* 20, no. 4 (June 7): 53–55.

Tomlinson, Tom, and Howard Brody. 1988. "Ethics and Communication in Do-not-Resuscitate Orders." *New England Journal of Medicine* 318, no. 1 (January 7): 43–46.

United States Catholic Conference. 1989. "USCC Brief in Nancy Cruzan Case." *Origins* 19, no. 21 (October 26): 345–51.

United States Conference of Catholic Bishops. 2001. *Ethical and Religious Directives for Catholic Health Care Services.* 4th ed. Washington, DC: United States Conference of Catholic Bishops.

U.S. Bishops' Pro-Life Committee. 1992. "Nutrition and Hydration: Moral and Pastoral Reflections." *Origins* 21, no. 44 (April 9): 705–12.

Vatican Information Service. 2004. "Patients in the Vegetative State Are Always Human." March 22.

Veatch, Robert M. 1973. "Generalization of Expertise." *Hastings Center Studies* 1 (2): 29–40.

Walter, James J. 2002. "Terminal Sedation: A Catholic Perspective." *Update* 18, no. 2 (September): 6–8.

Wear, Stephen, Benjamin Phillips, Sally Shimmel, and John Banas. 1995. "Developing and Implementing a Medical Futility Policy: One Hospital's Experience." *Community Ethics* 3, no. 1 (Winter): 2–5.

Wolf, Susan M. 1996. "Physician-Assisted Suicide in the Context of Managed Care." *Duquesne Law Review* 35, no. 1 (Fall): 455–79.

Wuerl, Donald W. 2005. "Reflection on Nutrition and Hydration." Bishop's statement.

Youngner, Stuart J. 1988. "Who Defines Futility?" *Journal of the American Medical Association* 260, no. 14 (October 14): 2094–95.

———. 1994. "Applying Futility: Saying No Is Not Enough." *Journal of the American Geriatrics Society* 42:887–89.

INDEX